SELECTED WORKS
OF
NATHAN FLAX

Volume 2

STRABISMUS & AMBLYOPIA

Optometric Extension Program Foundation, Inc.

Copyright © 2007 OEP Foundation, Inc.

The OEP Foundation, founded in 1928, is an international non-profit organization dedicated to continuing education and research for the advancement of human progress through education in behavioral vision care.

OEP Foundation, Inc.
1921 E. Carnegie Ave., Suite 3-L
Santa Ana, CA 92705
www.oep.org

Library of Congress Cataloging-in-Publication Data

Flax, Nathan.
    Selected works of Nathan Flax.
       p. cm.
    Includes bibliographical references (p.).
    Contents: v. 1. Case analysis, prescribing & treatment vision & learning -- v. 2. Strabismus & amblyopia.
ISBN 0-929780-11-6 (alk. Paper) vol. 1 --ISBN 0-929780-14-0 (alk. Paper) vol. 2

RE951.F55 2006
617.7'5--dc22
                                                                                                    2006051443

****

Optometry is the health care profession specifically licensed by state law to prescribe lenses, optical devices and procedures to improve human vision. Optometry has advanced vision therapy as a unique treatment modality for the development and remediation of the visual process. Effective vision therapy requires extensive understanding of:

- the effects of lenses (including prisms, filters and occluders)
- the variety of responses to the changes produced by lenses
- the various physiological aspects of the visual process
- the pervasive nature of the visual process in human behavior

As a consequence, effective vision therapy requires the supervision, direction and active involvement of the optometrist.

****

TABLE OF CONTENTS

STRABISMUS AND AMBLYOPIA

1. Introduction · 1
  Strabismus Diagnosis and Prognosis · 2

2. Strabismus Management · 21
  Brock's Techniques · 23
  New Concepts on the Control of Binocular Deviations · · · · · · · · · · · 27

3. Effectiveness of Visual Therapy · 32
  Orthoptic treatment of strabismus · 33

4. Intermittent Exotropia · 47
  Results of Surgical Treatment of Intermittent Divergent Strabismus · · · · · 48
  A Comparison of Functional Results In Intermittent Divergent Strabismus · · · · · · · 55
  Treated Surgically and Optometrically

5. A Treatment Approach for Divergence Excess Intermittent Exotropia · · · · · · · · 58
  The Optometric Training of Intermittent Divergent Strabismus · · · · · · · 59
  Training of Intermittent Exotropes · 65
  Management of Divergence Excess Intermittent Exotropia · · · · · · · · · · 73

6. Amblyopia · 77
  Pleoptics and Functional Optometry · 78
  Some Thoughts on the Clinical Management of Amblyopia · · · · · · · · · 83
  Common Sense Management of Amblyopia: Amblyopes are People, Not Eyes · · · · · · 88

STRABISMUS AND AMBLYOPIA

The paper on strabismus diagnosis and prognosis presented in this section was difficult to write. I had been asked to contribute a chapter for a text on vergence eye movements. Many of the chapters were to be authored by vision scientists working on the fundamental, basic mechanisms of vergence eye movements. My dilemma was to find the proper level of presentation so as to be informative for a sophisticated scientist uninvolved with clinical eye care, while at the same time useful to fellow optometric practitioners and students. It took a number of drafts before I found the correct "voice." I believe that this chapter meets the needs of both groups. While written more than 20 years ago, it is valid today.

The chapter, Strabismus and Prognosis, follows.

Strabismus Diagnosis and Prognosis

Nathan Flax
In: Schor C, Ciuffreda K, eds.
Vergence Eye Movements: Basic and Clinical Aspects.
Butterworths, 1983, 579-603
Reprinted with permission

Classification

Under normal circumstances, vergence movements maintain eye position so that there is foveal bifixation, with the visual axis deviating from the point of regard within the limits of fixation disparity - 30 minutes of arc or less. This rather precise positioning in individuals with normal binocular vision is mediated by a number of different vergence control mechanisms that have been classified by Maddox (1893) as tonic, accommodative, fusional, and proximal (Morgan, 1980). The net result of all the stimuli to vergence produces the precise motor response necessary to achieve bifoveal fixation, facilitating normal sensory integration of the two eyes.

In a substantial segment of the population there is failure to achieve or sustain such bifoveal alignment, resulting in the condition of strabismus (squint, tropia, or heterotropia). The incidence is most frequently reported as 2% to 3% of the population (Flom. 1963; Hugonnier and Hugonnier, 1969) but much higher figures are also given. The prevalence of strabismus is estimated in European studies at approximately 5.5% or 6% among six-year-olds (Graham, 1974). The National Center for Health Statistics of the United States Department of Health. Education and Welfare gives an incidence of 6.7% among children ages 6 to 17 (Roberts, 1972, 1975).

At first glance, clinical management of strabismus would seem to be simple and straightforward. If the eyes are not properly aligned, isolate the factor responsible and select an appropriate approach to relieve the condition. Unfortunately, this is far easier said than done. Few aspects of eye care are as complex and difficult as is the treatment of strabismus. Although the condition has been identified from earliest times (Revell, 1971), its etiology is often not known and controversy surrounds its treatment.

Strabismus is classified in a number of different ways. The various schemata are often based on different models that overlap and occasionally contradict one another. Nonetheless, all are useful in that they shed some light on the condition, contributing to the diagnosis and, more important, point the way to appropriate management. Several different classification schemata are discussed, with comments on their utility in establishing a diagnosis. This chapter is not directed toward detailed procedures for all available clinical techniques but rather deals selectively with a few that are illustrative and useful for understanding the problems of diagnosis and management of the strabismic patient. Numerous texts give specific procedures (Griffin, 1976; Hugonnier and Hugonnier, 1969; Burian and von Noorden, 1980).

Depending on facial configuration, shape of the orbital fissure, width of the nose, separation of the eyes, angle kappa (the angle between the line of sight and the perpendicular to the cornea at the center of the pupil), and other anatomic characteristics, two patients with identical angles of deviation may appear to have very different conditions. Wide noses with prominent epicanthal folds tend to increase the appearance of esotropia or mask exotropia. Most pseudostrabismus is due to the very prominent epicanthal folds of infancy, which create the impression of turn by reducing the amount of visible nasal sclera, particularly on lateral gaze when the iris of one eye may be partially obscured. High positive-angle kappas can give rise to the appearance of exotropia in patients who are actually not strabismic. This author has encountered the situation where successful therapy for childhood esotropia has resulted in the need to reassure the parents who were then suspicious of a divergent strabismus. A high-angle kappa had initially minimized the appearance of the convergent strabismus. After successful treatment achieved bifoveal fixation, there was the illusion of a small exotropia. While appearance does not bear any relationship to functional outcome, it is perhaps the most important consideration in the initiation of treatment.

The most frequently used classifications for strabismus are based on motor alignment of the eyes. Distinction is made between unilateral strabismus, in which one eye continually deviates, and alternating strabismus. The prognosis for ultimate functional cure is approximately the same in both cases (Flom, 1963], but other characteristics of the condition do relate to this distinction. The likelihood of amblyopia is minimal in alternators. Furthermore, if there is alternate fixation at distance there is strong likelihood of approximately equal refractive states in the two eyes. If the alternation occurs as a function of fixation distance, with one eye being used at distance and the other at near, the probability of anisometropia is high.

Direction of deviation is the next most obvious classification. Esotropes, exotropes, and hypertropes show different characteristics with decidedly different prognosis. As a group, exotropes are easier to cure than esotropes but generalizations are very difficult because of the influences of other factors. A rather high percentage of exotropes are intermittent and in this group, non-surgical functional cure rates are exceedingly high (Flax and Duckman, 1978). Esotropes tend to be constant and more difficult to treat functionally, particularly when anomalous retinal correspondence (ARC) is present (Flom, 1963). Hypertropia may involve a torsional component as well as elevation of an eye. In some instances, despite a small magnitude of deviation, functional results are difficult. Some vertical deviations can be compensated quite well with prism and show excellent results.

The angle of deviation is an important consideration, although not directly related to prognosis. There can be exceedingly high-angle esotropia with a large accommodative component, which can be well managed with convex lenses. Smaller angles of turn may be far more complex and resistant to treatment. Excellent results are achieved on intermittent exotropia of as much as 35 prism diopters, while poorer results sometimes occur in other patients who show anomalous retinal correspondence and constant esotropia of much smaller magnitude. Deviations of more than 35 prism diopters or less than 5 prism diopters tend to have a poorer functional prognosis (Flom, 1963).

An angle of turn that is constant in all directions of gaze is described as concomitant or comitant; an angle that varies as a function of the patient's direction of gaze is said to demonstrate lack of comitance or incomitance. Often incomitance is related to paralysis or paresis of one or more of the extra-ocular muscles, although anatomic abnormalities of the origin or insertion of a muscle, or of the orbital contents might also result in incomitance. In cases of paresis (or of hyperaction) of the extra-ocular muscles, the deficiency can be of the muscle itself or the innervations to the muscles. The classification of deviation by status of comitance does not give full insight into the condition. In some cases, such as a simple lateral rectus palsy, a patient may be left with perfectly intact binocular function in all fields of view except when the eyes move into the direction of action of the paralyzed muscle. The patient will be straight with bifoveal fixation on direct gaze but will demonstrate an increasing degree of esotropia when looking to the affected side. This condition may be a minimal handicap, since it is generally easy to compensate by turning the head or by suppressing vision of one eye on lateral gaze. Another patient with a similar involvement might not make a successful adaptation and consequently be bothered by intermittent diplopia. This patient may also suffer from asthenopia due to degradation of binocular function in the unaffected directions of gaze. Incomitance can take many forms and be of different degrees, ranging from inconsequential limitations of gaze on extreme version to significant limitation in or near primary gaze. Even minor muscle limitations can be disabling if they interfere with normal depression and convergence necessary for reading.

Still another diagnostic classification is the variability of turn angle. It is important to know if the angle of turn changes from one moment to the next and the conditions that precipitate change. It is not unusual for parents to report that a child's eyes appear straighter at the beginning of the day and more turned toward the end of the day or when the youngster is fatigued, ill, or emotionally upset. In other instances there is a variability in angle that does not relate to any specific time of day, state of fatigue, or particular task demand. A turn angle that varies as a function of detail of target or distance of fixation is suspicious of an accommodative component. Careful case history and repeated examination may be necessary to understand properly the fluctuations. One common circumstance that introduces variability is the distance of the fixation target. This change in motor status may be related to refractive considerations. This will be discussed later.

Strabismus can also be classified based on the frequency of deviation. A turn may be constant or intermittent. If intermittent, its occurrence may vary from occasional to frequent. It is generally not difficult to differentiate an intermittent from a constant strabismus at time of examination unless there is variability related to fatigue or time of day. Under such circumstance the patient might show a constant strabismus late in the day and an intermittent turn if examined earlier. Case history data are useful and important in making this distinction.

From a therapeutic point of view, frequency of turn is an exceedingly important consideration. It would seem to be unwise, for instance, to choose surgical interference, with its attendant risks, for a strabismic condition that appears only infrequently. Occasional turns have excellent functional prognosis with appropriate orthoptic therapy (Flom, 1963). The presence of any degree of intermittency improves the prognosis greatly as it implies some basis for normal function at least part of the time and a high probability of a functional neuro-sensory system. Careful and provocative testing is required to distinguish properly between a constant turn of variable angle and a true intermittent strabismus. Often, parental reports in this regard are misleading. It is possible for a child to be constantly strabismic, yet have an angle that varies from cosmetically acceptable to noticeable. This is often construed by parents as a shift from straight to turn. The prognostic implications are quite different when there is, in fact, bifoveal fixation at least part of the time as contrasted to a constant strabismus with an angle that reduces to cosmetically acceptable limits on occasion. In the latter case, intactness of neuro-sensory function cannot be assumed. When this author encounters such a situation and suspects that the parental report of straight eyes has actually been a response to a reduction in angle of deviation, the parents are brought into the examination routine and asked to assess eye position by their criteria so that the history can be properly interpreted.

Age of onset of strabismus is another important classification. It is highly desirable to ascertain whether it is congenital or acquired. Unfortunately, this is not always easily determined. It is generally accepted that congenital strabismus has a far more dismal prognosis insofar as functional binocularity is concerned, and it can also have a profound influence on amblyopia. Animal experiments point to critical periods very early in life that are vital to establishment and maintenance of the underlying neurology to permit clear central acuity. Animals deprived of form vision during the critical stages of neurological development suffer irreparable loss of acuity together with demonstrable neural changes. Deprivation before and after a critical period produces functional deficits that are largely reversible with appropriate stimulation (Blakemore, 1974; Van Sluyters, 1978). Just exactly how to apply this research in humans is not fully clear. By consensus rather than experimental evidence it is usually assumed that humans have a somewhat longer and probably less critical "critical period" than do the animals studied. Most feel that acuity development in children is highly susceptible to deprivation up to the age of three or three and one half years. This has led to reconsideration of the role of early correction of refractive error (particularly astigmatism and anisometropia) in the interest of providing clear imagery during the sensitive period (Ikeda and Wright, 1975; Mitchell et al., 1973). Some difficulties in clinical management are not fully resolved. It would seem desirable fully to correct ametropia in very young children; however, refraction is not stable in infancy. Rapid changes in astigmatism, for instance, are normal in the first year or so of life (Atkinson et al., 1980; Mohindra et al., 1978).

Clinical decisions are not easy to make. Where there is high astigmatism or high anisometropia, the need to provide clear focus on the retina almost seems to demand refractive correction. The question must be raised about the impact of high anisometropic correction on fusion due to problems of aniseikonia (image size) that may be created, and the introduction of variable prismatic stimulation to vergence. Is there the possibility that therapy to minimize the probability of amblyopia may have an adverse effect on fusion? The same question may be raised regarding the use of occlusion therapy in early strabismus. Not only does occluding an eye in a very young infant carry the risk of development of occlusion amblyopia in a previously sound eye (Burian, 1966; Ikeda and Wright, 1975; Thomas et al., 1979), the deprivation associated with early occlusion may in fact reduce the potential for later fusion. In animal experiments, reduction of the number of binocularly driven cortical cells as a function of occlusion during critical periods is well established (Blakemore, 1976; Hubel and Wiesel, 1965). Just how this relates to sensory fusion or motor control of the eyes in humans is speculative, but at very least it offers reason to be more cautious in the use of occlusion in infants. In general, it is accepted that congenital strabismics do not show a very hopeful prognosis for normal binocular function. Acquired strabismus of late onset generally has a good binocular function prognosis. Just where the transition line is remains to be established.

There are other important aspects of onset. Long-standing strabismus generally presents a different clinical picture than that of more recent onset. If its basis is a paretic ocular muscle, the specific offending muscle becomes far more difficult to detect with the passage of time. The motor deficiency tends to spread into other areas of gaze and becomes generalized (Burian and von Noorden, 1980). This is both good and bad. It complicates specific motor diagnosis but it may offer a more functionally useful motor system because a deviation that is consistent in all fields of gaze is easier to compensate by head-turning or use of a prism correction, and therefore may enhance the prognosis. Sensory concomitants of strabismus (which will be dealt with in some detail later in this chapter) such as diplopia, suppression, or anomalous retinal correspondence may change with the passage of time so that the functional status of a longtime strabismus may be quite different from one of recent onset. Sudden onset is highly suspicious of pathology, and must be investigated.

Another classification in diagnosis has to do with etiology. There are several potential causes of strabismus ranging from anatomic or mechanical interferences with eye movement because of congenital malformation or trauma, to functional or innervational abnormalities. It is desirable to ascertain etiology, although data in this regard are minimal and generally of questionable reliability. All too often investigation of the problem is done long after initial onset, making it difficult to establish clearly both time of onset and specific etiology.

The refractive state of the patient frequently relates to strabismus and becomes an important part of diagnosis. There are two different ways in which it relates to strabismus. One has to do with the direct influence of accommodative convergence on the alignment of the eyes. The other concerns influence of ametropia, particularly anisometropia, on sensory fusion processes. A frequent cause is uncorrected hyperopia, particularly in the presence of a high AC/A ratio. The accommodative effort necessary to compensate for the hyperopia induces so great an accommodative convergence response that the fusional vergence capability of the patient is overwhelmed, resulting in a loss of alignment. Typically, such strabismus develops fairly early in life, although later onset is possible. As a rule, accommodative esotropia is first noted at near, where the influence of accommodative convergence is greatest. In higher amounts of hyperopia (or in lower amounts with a high AC/A ratio) the squint may be present at all fixation distances. An important part of diagnostic evaluation involves ascertaining the influence of accommodation on the turn angle. The presence of a significant AC/A linkage in any strabismus, convergent or divergent, has a profound influence on therapeutic strategy and eventual outcome. A high ratio permits excellent leverage with use of lenses and should suggest caution when surgery is contemplated; the same high AC/A that may have precipitated a strabismus can be harnessed through lenses to assist in diverging the eyes. Failure to allow properly for an accommodative component can lead to post surgical disaster. This writer has encountered patients with high AC/A ratios who were operated "successfully," only to have difficulty when it became necessary at a later date to correct existing hyperopia to alleviate asthenopia. Application of corrective lenses induced exotropia in a patient who had been esotropic before the surgery. Asthenopia and/or recurrence of the turn are generally avoidable consequences if the AC/A influence is appropriately planned for.

Refraction has an indirect influence on strabismus by virtue of its influence on the sensory processes of binocular vision. High astigmatism can cause amblyopia that degrades fusion. In an individual with high heterophoria this can become a factor in the manifestation of squint. Perhaps the most serious refractive interference to sensory fusion is that caused by anisometropia. Under normal circumstances it is assumed that the accommodative levels of the two eyes are the same and determined by the fixing eye. In uncorrected anisometropia it is not possible for the patient to maintain clear vision in each eye simultaneously (except possibly for special conditions of marked asymmetric convergence) (Rosenberg et al., 1953). If the eyes possess different degrees of hyperopia, the usual response is for the eye with the lower refractive state to set the binocular accommodative response, leaving the eye with the greater hyperopia continually blurred. This leads to amblyopia of the more ametropic eye, and in turn, produces confusion of clear and blurred images both appearing to be located in the same place, setting the stage for suppression. Suppression reduces the effectiveness of fusional vergence and contributes to squint. In myopic anisometropia, or when one eye is hyperopic and the other eye myopic, several possibilities exist depending on the degree of anisometropia. In milder cases the least myopic eye or the hyperopic eye may become dominant for distance and the more myopic eye dominant for near tasks. In such situations suppression is present although amblyopia is rare. If, however, the more myopic eye shows very high myopia, it may be suppressed at all distances with accompanying amblyopia. Exotropia and deep amblyopia of a highly myopic and anisometropic eye are not unusual.

Occasionally, strabismus may be due to deprivation because of early cataract or blindness in one eye. The latter condition traditionally has had a very poor prognosis but recent work with eye movement and biofeedback techniques offer the hope of straightening a blind eye (Goldrich, 1982; Hirons and Yolton, 1978).

There are two types of strabismus that involve a significant change in deviation. One is an exotropia that occurs past childhood or in old age following long-standing esotropia and the second is a post surgical strabismus. Both have a guarded prognosis for functional binocularity.

There is one classification scheme for strabismus that is frequently used and with which this author disagrees. This is the use of the terms "latent" and "manifest" deviation. Some authors treat phoria and strabismus conditions as being essentially the same thing. They categorize by direction of deviation and differentiate between the two by classifying phoria as a latent strabismus and strabismus as opposed to manifest overt strabismus. This tends to minimize an exceedingly important distinction between them. Strabismus describes the condition whereby the two visual axes do not aim at a common point of regard when there is no artificial impediment to binocular vision. A phoria is an artificially produced circumstance in which fusional vergence cues are either not available or diplopic images are optically separated by so great an amount as to exceed any reasonable vergence capacity. Under these conditions the eyes deviate to a vergence position dictated by all of the Maddox innervations except fusion. In strabismus the eyes deviate despite the fact that the stimulus array contains cues that ordinarily permit a normal vergence mechanism to produce alignment. This is not to say that all strabismus is due to faulty fusional vergence, since there can be other considerations that preclude alignment. The important issue is that phorias and strabismus actually represent a significant change of state. Despite this, many authors lump the two together on the basis of the direction of deviation. Esodeviations and exodeviations are discussed and both phorias and strabismus included under one heading. Even surgical results are sometimes presented this way, a practice that this author feels is unwarranted and confusing (Burian and von Noorden, 1980).

Adaptations

Motor-based schemata are not sufficient to diagnose strabismus. Appropriate management requires understanding of the sensory aspects of the condition as well. As a consequence of the failure of a strabismic to align both eyes, the object of regard is imaged on the fovea of the fixing eye and some off-foveal point in the deviating eye. For the strabismic patient with normal retinal correspondence these two stimulated points do not give rise to the perception of common visual directions. This results in diplopia unless some compensatory mechanism is invoked.

Suppression, the disappearance from consciousness of one image, is a frequent adaptive response to restore single vision. Suppression of a diplopically seen image does not involve the fovea of the deviated eye, but rather the off-foveal point in the eye that receives the same image as the fovea of the fixing eye.

Foveal suppression occurs for a different reason. Under normal circumstances the two foveas share a common subjective visual direction. Objects imaged on them are perceived as being located at the same place. In the absence of ocular alignment the two foveas carry images of different objects. Two different things would appear to occupy the same position in space. This "confusion" is a more disabling condition than is diplopia of a single object and hence there is suppression of data associated with the fovea of the deviated eye. The perception of two things in the same place is apparently so disturbing to overall function that it is a rare symptom. Patient reports of confusion are so infrequent as to indicate that suppression of the foveal image of the deviated eye probably occurs at the moment of turn. Even intermittent strabismics, who rather often experience diplopia, almost never report confusion. Diplopia can apparently be lived with more successfully and is more often reported. This author has encountered young patients with long-standing diplopia who never told anyone of it because they felt that "everyone saw that way." They reported a real-unreal distinction (McLaughlin, 1964) that permitted them to reach successfully for door knobs and the like. They used the preferred image for guiding movement and were surprisingly little bothered by the second "false" image. This is generally not the case in adult strabismics of recent onset who find it difficult or impossible to adapt to the diplopia.

Theoretical discussion of suppression makes it sound more constant an entity than it actually is. The suppression scotomas of the fovea and the off-foveal points discussed in the preceding paragraphs are not nearly as discrete as might be expected. In clinical testing suppression is most often an amorphous, continually shifting and changing phenomenon that is very much influenced by intensity of attention and variation in stimulus conditions. Brightness, color, size, and movement of stimulus have profound influence over what is suppressed and when. Suppressed objects can appear and disappear, wax and wane, as attention is directed to them, or their stimulus value changed by modification of the target or its surround. Merely changing ambient illumination or jiggling the target is often sufficient to overcome suppression and permit diplopia awareness. A small muscle light may be suppressed where a slightly larger bulb may be seen double. A red lens before the deviating eye can produce diplopia awareness and even the density of the red filter can influence suppression. Using a bell to add noise to the visual target or having the patient touch the target can reduce or eliminate suppression. Suppression by strabismics may also be a function of viewing distance, direction of gaze, refractive correction, and target detail. It is an elusive, variable, but often useful adaptation to strabismus.

Another sensory adaptation is anomalous retinal correspondence (ARC). While most frequently considered as a consequence, there is also the possibility that ARC can sometimes be the cause of deviation. This point of view has been offered, but most prevailing opinions are that anomalous correspondence follows rather than precedes deviation. In ARC the two foveas do not share common subjective visual directions. Rather, the fovea of one eye shares a common direction with an off-foveal point in the other eye. In harmonious ARC the corresponding retinal points are the fovea of the fixing eye and the point in the deviated eye that receives the same stimulus. This is a very utilitarian situation. There is no stimulus to diplopia. There could still be two areas of "clear" vision, one viewed by the fixing eye and one of some peripheral place where the fovea of the deviating eye happens to be pointed, but no confusion would exist since this clear image would be appreciated as peripheral to the point of regard (Brock, 1945; Cooper and Feldman, 1979).

Harmonious ARC would seem to be a most sensible adaptation to a motor deviation. The angle of anomaly, the angle between the. subjective directionalization of the two foveas, is equal to the angle of turn and therefore the subjective angle of turn is zero. In effect the patient recalibrates sensory correspondence exactly to neutralize the angle of turn. Diplopia is avoided, both eyes can contribute to spatial judgments, and there may even be a bonus of a secondary area of clear vision in the field of view. Stereoacuity is reduced, but gross peripheral stereopsis is often demonstrated. Typically, a patient with harmonious ARC (HARC) is but little handicapped in normal environments. There is generally absence of asthenopia; there is no diplopia. Distance judgments are frequently quite accurate, particularly in a complex environment where decisions are not limited solely to disparity detection. Patients park automobiles in tight spaces successfully and this author has seen some who are highly skilled at hitting and catching a baseball.

While it is true that some patients with HARC (as well as many with monolateral strabismus and deep amblyopia) become remarkably adept at using monocular distance and depth cues in normal environments, most also use binocular cues in daily life. This is easily demonstrated by occluding the deviated eye. In monolateral strabismus with suppression this maneuver has little impact on performance. In HARC cases, covering the turned eye degrades performance on the Brock stick-in-straw test (Brock, 1956) in much the same way that it does for normals. This can sometimes be used as a diagnostic test for young patients incapable of response to more sophisticated tests. Noticeable degradation of spatial and depth judgment skills with turned eye covered is suggestive of HARC.

Harmonious ARC is a logical adaptive concomitant strabismus. Covariation of the angle of anomaly and the angle of deviation would seem to support this notion (Hallden, 1952). Presence of ARC while deviated and normal retinal correspondence (NRC) when aligned among intermittent strabismics (Cooper and Feldman, 1979) and the generally accepted clinical impression that among esotropes ARC is most likely to be demonstrated under circumstances closely relating to daily life and least likely to be manifested under circumstances remote from daily life are also consistent with this premise (Burian, 1951; Griffin, 1976; Burian and von Noorden, 1980). Unfortunately, like most things associated with strabismus, the problem of ARC is not always as cleanly dealt with as this discussion would imply. Not all patients show covariation. Of those who do, the covariation is not always precisely correlated to maintain mathematical equality of the objective angle of turn and the angle of anomaly (Kerr, 1969). Not all intermittent strabismics show the pattern of ARC while deviated and NRC while aligned. Not all ARC patients are harmonious.

Nonharmonious ARC (NHARC) presents a theoretical conundrum. There is an angle of anomaly other than zero but the angle of anomaly and angle of turn are not equal. This leaves the patient with a type of correspondence that is neither normal nor functional. Subjective and objective angles of turn do not agree but the functional advantage of this is not apparent. The patient with NHARC still has to suppress to avoid diplopia. Harmonious ARC is logical and useful; NHARC seems to have little purpose other than to complicate diagnosis and treatment. Several explanations are offered for the presence of NHARC. One is that the squint angle had been different at some prior time in the patient's life and that HARC developed as a compensation. Then something suddenly changed the angle of turn, leaving the patient with NHARC (Burian, 1945). This is plausible in some instances, particularly those in which surgical intervention has changed the angle of turn. A second explanation supposes that there is a gradual shift of NRC to HARC but that the adaptive process has not been sufficient to change the correspondence fully to match the squint angle (Ronne and Rindziunski, 1953). This author has great difficulty in accepting this line of reasoning. For such a process to occur there would have to be some positive reinforcement as the retinal correspondence shifted away from NRC toward HARC. No such reward exists since there is no patient benefit in terms of function in daily life from anything other than complete elimination of the subjective angle. In-between stages might actually be disadvantageous since they would shift a diplopic image (if there were no suppression) from the periphery toward the point of fixation, a situation that would seem to be more difficult to cope with than widely separated images.

There are several explanations offered for the physiological mechanisms whereby ARC is produced. Hallden (1952) proposed a sensory process in which retinal correspondence changes are independent of motor movements of the eyes. Morgan (1961) offers a theory of "registered" eye movements that produce change in retinal correspondence. These registered movements may be due to non-accommodative vergence innervation. Kerr (1980) ascribes this to neurologically defective fusional vergence control. This might explain NHARC, since no purposeful adaptation is implied in this theory.

Another aspect of ARC that bears on diagnosis and management of strabismus is the variability of response in a single subject. It is possible for some patients to shift from normal to anomalous correspondence on the basis of a change in vergence angle or in various aspects of a stimulus array including size of target detail. Most fascinating is the condition wherein a patient exhibits ARC and NRC simultaneously. This phenomenon, called binocular triplopia, can sometimes be elicited in a major amblyoscope with first-degree targets placed at the objective angle. With flashing or oscillation of the targets and use of suggestion, it is sometimes possible for patients to view one of the targets in two different localizations simultaneously; one according to normal binocular projection and the other localized anomalously (Burian and von Noorden, 1980; Griffin, 1976). When this therapeutic procedure is used, the anomalous image fades from view; it does not shift position toward the normal image. This response pattern is not consistent with the hypotheses of a gradual shift of retinal correspondence from normal to anomalous.

Generally, ARC is felt to be a response to the misalignment of the eyes. The reverse situation cannot be dismissed completely, for if ARC was "wired in" then strabismus would result as a logical consequence. A patient with anatomically fixed ARC would seek strabismus in much the same way that normals seek alignment. Irregularities in retinal correspondence across the field of view are cited by Flom (1980) to explain some of the behaviors associated with strabismus. Regardless of whether or not ARC is the cause or effect of strabismus, its presence in any case other than intermittent exotropia complicates therapy. Congenital strabismics with consistent ARC on all tests almost always defy treatment to normalize correspondence.

In view of the complexities of both suppression and retinal correspondence, the diagnostic routine should include a variety of tests of each so as to ascertain the patient's sensory status over a range of different stimulus conditions. Each of the functions can and does change, in some instances, as a function of the particular test probe used (Burian and von Noorden, 1980; Griffin, 1976). Another sensory aspect of strabismus has to do with the patient's fusion capability. Worth (1921) described three aspects of binocular integration that he labeled first, second, and third degrees. Some patients are capable of first-degree integration or simultaneous awareness of inputs of each eye in the absence of fusable contours. Other patients can effect true sensory integration of second-degree targets, which requires coalescing of similar inputs from each eye into a single percept. Still others are capable of stereopsis (Worth's third-degree fusion). To probe these functions the test materials must either be presented at the crossing point of the visual axes in the case of esotropes or by use of optically dissociated stimuli along the line of sight of each eye. This latter technique can be accomplished by use of a Wheatstone or a Brewster stereoscope, or anaglyphs or vectograms.

As in so many other areas of strabismus work, some of the apparently obvious considerations do not necessarily pertain. It is erroneous, for instance, to think of simultaneous awareness, second-degree fusion (flat fusion), and third-degree fusion (stereopsis) as representing some sort of continuum in ascending order. This is not necessarily so. In a normal environment it is all but impossible to encounter first-degree stimulus conditions, and second-degree stimulus conditions are rare. There are almost always disparity cues available in real life situations. It requires careful manipulation of inputs to achieve first- or second - degree conditions. As a consequence, there are some strabismic patients who do better with third-degree fusion stimuli. Failure on a first-degree target does not preclude successful appreciation of a stereoscopic target. Diagnostic testing should include all three types of probes. Some strabismics, particularly intermittent exotropes, can at times maintain bifoveal alignment and demonstrate binocular integration more readily when presented with stereoscopic demands than when asked to deal with first-degree or second-degree stimuli (Flax, 1963; Goldrich, 1980).

Still another factor that must be checked is the capacity to make fusional vergence responses. If the patient is able to demonstrate second-or third-degree fusion either at a centration point in finite space where the visual axes cross or at the angle of deviation in a stereoscopic instrument, it is necessary to find out the patient's capacity to change the angle of deviation in response to a fusional vergence demand. This should be probed in both the converging and diverging directions from the angle of turn. Presence of a fusional vergence response, however slight, offers a favorable prognosis for ultimate binocular cure. In the case of an esotrope it is important to determine whether or not there is a centration range over which the eyes change vergence angle to achieve bifoveal fixation, regardless of how close to the patient this range might be. It is also useful to see if binocular alignment is triggered by a spatial manipulation task, such as placing a stick into a straw (which is held by the examiner in such a way that the task requires a depth judgment rather than aiming). This is sometimes the situation in near-point exotropes who do not converge just to look at a target but who will converge and bifoveally fixate when asked to make a spatial judgment that cannot be made accurately other than by use of either triangulation or stereoscopic data. The presence of such a positive response is a favorable indicator.

While motor and sensory factors are related, the linkage is not always consistent or predictable. Angle of turn does not necessarily correlate with magnitude or sensory impairment. Patients with small angle turns are not by definition more normal in function than those with larger angles of deviation. It is possible to find a patient with a large deviation who shows normal retinal correspondence, and another patient with a smaller turn angle with anomalous correspondence. Which is more normal? Does a patient with minimum motor deviation who is not capable of sensory fusion represent a greater or lesser departure from normal than another patient with a large angular deviation who can demonstrate a normal sensory relationship, including stereopsis, under appropriate stimulus conditions? It is even possible for an individual with strabismus to demonstrate more "normal" binocular function than does one with perfect alignment. For instance, one criterion of binocular vision is stereopsis. Yet there are non-strabismics who have poor or no stereopsis (Movshon et al., 1972; Richards, 1969), while some with strabismus can demonstrate excellent stereoacuity so long as the disparity is presented in such a manner that the inputs are along the lines of sight of each eye.

There are situations in which patients who are strabismic may perform in a complex environment in a manner more efficient than others who do not have strabismus. For instance, in the condition variously labeled monofixational phoria (Parks, 1964), microtropia (Lang, 1968), or monofixational syndrome (Parks, 1969), there is misalignment of the visual axes in the order of 2 to 10 prism diopters with absence of bifoveal fixation, yet the patients will usually demonstrate fairly sophisticated functional binocularity. Such patients can show peripheral fusion (Burian, 1941) and stereopsis. They generally appear cosmetically straight and the turn is frequently not detected by the cover test, which is usually the most effective means of diagnosing the presence of strabismus. Patients with microtropia may fare better at daily tasks than non-strabismics, who by virtue of a different type of binocular dysfunction, demonstrate frequent suppression or inadequate motor fusion ranges. Despite the fact that the eyes are straight in terms of motor function, the non-strabismics may have asthenopia whereas the microtropics characteristically do not experience discomfort.

Some of the sensory concomitants of strabismus serve adaptive purposes. Harmonious ARC is functionally quite useful in normal environments. Suppression can eliminate diplopia or confusion and permit the strabismic patient to operate very well in daily life despite the absence of bifoveal fusion. Many people become quite adept at using so-called monocular cues to make spatial and depth judgments. Strabismic patients do not see a flat world; they see a three-dimensional world, although they are not always capable of normal stereopsis. At times the handicap can be small, there being poor correlation between degree of strabismus caused impairment in binocular function and difficulty in daily life. At times there may even be a negative correlation. Lesser degrees of binocular dysfunction may have greater impact on daily tasks than do greater dysfunctions. This writer has frequently encountered intermittent esotropes or moderate esophores who were asthenopic, in contrast to constant esotropes who have adapted successfully through suppression or ARC and showed minimal difficulty in normal activities. Intermittent strabismics would certainly have to be considered to have a higher degree of binocular function than constant strabismics, and yet this does not necessarily mean that the former are more comfortable or efficient. Using a grading scale based on the usual criteria of binocular vision, they would have to be rated as being better visually than their counterparts who show constant strabismus. Yet when faced with sustaining attention at reading they appear to be far more disabled than the constantly strabismic patient. This is an issue that has never been dealt with adequately in research studies and confounds the relationship between vision and academic performance (Flax, 1970; Spache, 1976).

Similarly, while the suppression amblyopia of strabismus certainly represents a serious visual deficiency, under ordinary circumstances it has less impact on daily function than might be anticipated. Suppression, by eliminating confusion or diplopia, may facilitate performance, particularly if the task can be accomplished without use of stereopsis cues. Suppression amblyopia degrades stereoacuity, but most tasks do not require fine stereopsis. The patient with amblyopia tends to have consistent (albeit reduced) binocular input, permitting reasonable performance, sometimes more so than a patient with a lesser degree of suppression who must deal with continually changing ocular inputs.

This author feels there is insufficient attention given to the relationship of the strabismic condition to performance. Most often the analysis of departure from clinical norms, emphasizing angle of turn or various aspects of binocular vision, pays scant attention to the impact of the ocular misalignment on the patient's ability to function out of the examination room. Treatment options are evaluated primarily in terms of the binocular measures and rarely consider overall performance, although this is actually more important than the binocular skills themselves.

Testing

While it is not the intent of this chapter to discuss specific tests used in strabismus diagnosis, some comment is in order, particularly in view of the increased interest in early detection and diagnosis. In many instances the angle of turn is sufficiently large so that there is no question as to the presence of the condition. In other cases the turn angle may be small and the ocular and facial configurations such that strabismus is not readily apparent. With a cooperative patient the best single method to ascertain the presence of strabismus is the cover test. Successful application of this procedure requires that the patient be willing and able to maintain attention on a small target. Very young infants are captured by a bright and novel target presented at close distances and it is therefore possible to obtain satisfactory measurement at near, but it is exceedingly difficult to test at further distances. Older infants are particularly difficult to assess by cover tests, since it is not always possible to be sure that they are directing their attention as the examiner would like.

The presence of central fixation (or stable, consistent eccentric fixation) is another necessary condition for an accurate cover test. Demonstration of normal visual acuity can be taken as evidence of central fixation. Unfortunately, this is not always testable in infants and young children by usual clinical methods. When visual acuity can be measured, the presence of amblyopia should make the examiner suspicious of eccentric fixation. It is not an absolute indicator, however, since amblyopia can exist even with central fixation. There are several fairly refined procedures to ascertain the presence of eccentric fixation using entopic phenomenona, such as the Haidinger brush or the Maxwell spot, which subjectively tag the directional locus of the fovea in space, but these require reasonably sophisticated patient responses (Ludlam, 1970). It is also possible to place the fovea under direct observation using a projection type ophthalmoscope that presents targets visible to both patient and examiner. This technique does not require the patient to describe a weakly perceived phenomenon such as a Maxwell spot or Haidinger brush, but does call for patient cooperation to the point of being able to participate actively (Burian and von Noorden, 1980). Infants will aim their eyes at a bright light such as presented with an ophthalmoscope but young children at times can be notoriously uncooperative. Certain at-risk populations, such as children with brain injury or cerebral palsy, who show high instances of strabismus and amblyopia are frequently unable to participate in this type of testing (Duckman, 1979; Harcourt, 1974). While larger degrees of eccentricity can be detected by observing the first Purkinje image of a muscle light, smaller degrees of eccentric fixation are all but impossible to detect with certainty in an uncooperative patient.

When the cover test cannot be applied it becomes necessary to rely on Purkinje image location to assess the presence and magnitude of strabismus. By means of a muscle light the location of the cornea reflection is noted in each eye under two-eyed viewing conditions. Asymmetry of the image location is assumed to be due to strabismus and the magnitude of asymmetry is a measure of the angle of the strabismus deviation. This Hirshberg method has been in use for many years. It is generally rather poorly specified so that converting the linear displacement of the corneal reflex to an angular measurement is fairly crude. For many years it was generally assumed that 1mm displacement of reflected image represented 13 prism diopters of deviation (Morgan, 1963). Flom (1956) offered a formula that took into account the nonlinearity of the measurement, improving the accuracy of the Hirshberg test. Recently there have been several attempts systematically to compare Hirshberg estimates of squint angle to actual measurement of the deviation. This has produced a surprising result indicating that, on average, 1 mm displacement of the corneal light reflex equals approximately 22 prism diopters of angular deviation (Jones and Eskridge, 1970). Griffin and Boyer (1974) found that in individual patients 1 mm of corneal light reflex displacement varied from as little as 9.4 to as much as 68.2 prism diopters of deviation. In view of the enormous interest in early diagnosis and intervention it is ironic that so much of the clinical literature hinges on such crude measurements. Accurate determination of the existence and magnitude of small-angle strabismus in infants is based on fleeting observation and assumption of where the infant is in fact directing attention, and a crude method of interpreting the location of the corneal light reflex. Additionally, the use of a light as a stimulus does not afford good control over accommodative level.

There are many elegant tests for retinal correspondence and fusion (Griffin, 1976; Hugonnier and Hugonnier, 1969; Ludlam, 1970). Unfortunately, most are difficult if not impossible to use successfully with infants and young children. They all require subjective responses and a degree of cooperation not always present in preschoolers. In many cases the young child, highly suggestible and anxious to please the examiner, responds to other than visual cues when confronted with a confusing and demanding test circumstance. Use of objective tests such as visually evoked potentials (Amigo et al., 1978), elimination of ambiguity in testing by random-dot stereograms (Cooper and Feldman, 1978a; Reinecke and Simons, 1974), or behavior modification techniques (Cooper and Feldman, 1978b) all can serve to assist in permitting more accurate diagnosis of young children. Unfortunately, the number of procedures that have been developed thus far is relatively small and not all diagnostic areas can be tapped without reasonably sophisticated cooperation.

Prognosis

The ultimate purpose of diagnosis is to arrive at a prognosis and a decision as to management. Many factors must be considered, of which perhaps the most important is cosmetic appearance. That this is so is attested to by the frequency of strabismus surgery as a therapeutic measure, despite the generally poor functional results. Multiple surgeries are frequent and reported functional cure rates vary widely, some as low as 10% (Ludlam, 1970). Burian and von Noorden (1980) report two series of congenital esotropes involving 100 patients in which 159 operations produced straight eyes, and the possibility of normal binocular function in only seven patients.

Data regarding functional cures with surgery must be carefully analyzed since, in this author's opinion, most studies are seriously flawed either by inclusion of minimal success criteria or by non-identification of criteria. Perhaps the most egregious deficiency is the use of success standards that were probably present in the patients before surgery. This is exemplified in a summary of 775 cases of operations for exodeviation (Burian and von Noorden, 1980). Inspection of the cited papers discloses such deficiencies as including intermittent exotropes who might have met the success criteria prior to operation (Burian and Spivey, 1965); using presence of stereopsis as a cure criterion in a sample comprised solely of intermittent exotropes (Pratt-Johnson et al., 1977), despite the fact that most intermittent exotropes show stereopsis when aligned (Cooper, 1977); treating half of the sample orthoptically in addition to surgery and accepting any degree of stereopsis as a functional result (Hardesty et al., 1978); ignoring near point function or alignment as criteria of satisfactory results while restricting the sample to patients who demonstrated fusion and stereopsis before surgery (Ballen, 1970); using alignment on cover test as an indication of binocular function with no tests for fusion or stereopsis (Windsor, 1971); or requiring fusion capability including stereopsis before operation, considering reduction of the deviation to within 10Δ of straight as a success, and ignoring residual near deviations (Raab and Parks, 1969). The approximate 50% aggregate success really represents cosmetic improvement rather than functional cure.

Elimination of functional deficiencies in binocular vision, performance difficulties, and asthenopia should be considered in addition to cosmetic appearance. When feasible, this author considers orthoptics to be the preferred treatment (along with refractive correction and/or prisms). Inasmuch as the major emphasis in orthoptics is establishment of normal sensory fusion in order ultimately to effect alignment of the eyes, the approach is preferred to surgery. Unless surgery completely eliminates the strabismus it cannot be expected to have a significant impact on function. Even a slight residual misalignment of the eyes creates a situation that causes diplopia or requires functional adaptation by suppression or development of anomalous retinal correspondence. The adage "a miss is as good as a mile" must be kept in mind when relating functional outcomes with surgery. While it may infrequently result in normal retinal correspondence, this cannot be depended on (Burian and von Noorden, 1980). Thus it should be the back-up to orthoptics, not the other way around, since when feasible, orthoptics can produce more functional cures. Flax and Duckman (1978) reporting on 928 cases in 12 studies with well-stated, high-level success criteria, found 67% cure in orthoptics supervised by ophthalmologists and 86% cure when the orthoptic treatment was done by optometrists. Cosmetic surgery is always an option if functional results are not possible.

Optical limitations should be evaluated prior to undertaking therapy. For instance, if there is anisometropia, the introduction of possible anisophoria or aniseikonic difficulties must be considered. Hindrance to fusion may be caused by the variable prism induced by anisometropic spectacles. The cosmetic aspects of an anisometropic correction must also be considered. While contact lenses frequently are desirable, it must be established that the patient will tolerate them. In some instances it might be desirable to treat the strabismus by developing peripheral fusion to effect alignment and reasonably good binocular function without correcting the anisometropic refraction. In certain instances it is conceivable that full anisometropic correction may create more difficulties than benefits. Along the same line, the patient's potential fusional capabilities should be determined before undertaking treatment. In situations in which no fusion can be demonstrated under any circumstances during evaluation or, more particularly, in situations where horror fusionis is demonstrated, any therapeutic regimen should proceed very cautiously (Griffin, 1976). It is relatively easy to eliminate suppression; it is all but impossible to teach a patient to suppress. The best that can be done in situations of intractable diplopia is to use optical blur or occlusion in the hope of the patient developing suppression. This is not always successful. The possibility of asthenopia on conclusion of treatment should be considered if the optical and fusional factors indicate that at best, very tenuous or weak fusion might be achieved. The patient might best be treated in a manner not designed to introduce an uncomfortable situation. Thoughtless pursuit of a particular therapeutic objective at the expense of the patient's well-being is not desirable. For instance, one occasionally encounters a youngster who has been occluded for years in an attempt to improve an amblyopic eye, with total disregard of the effect of occlusion on the youngster's overall development. Methods of restraining a youngster from removing an eye patch are discussed (Hiles and Galket, 1974) with little concern about the effects on general performance and emotional well being of a child forced to function using a significantly amblyopic eye for an extended period of time with full knowledge that he or she possesses an eye that can see properly.

Heroic attempts to establish binocular alignment in cerebral palsied children may be ill advised. Many of these patients have great difficulty in successfully developing the usual functional adaptations that permit other strabismic children to perform. This author has encountered children with cerebral palsy who habitually fixated with the more amblyopic eye, turning what seemed to be the more functionally useful eye. Considering their multiple handicaps, including a high incidence of oculomotor dysfunction, one must carefully consider whether the surgical treatment of a strabismus is not possibly more harmful than beneficial, particularly in view of a very poor functional prognosis (Harcourt, 1974).

There are numerous factors that offer a favorable prognosis. Full and comitant motor capability is obviously an excellent prognostic sign. An accommodative component in esotropia or the ability to use accommodative convergence as a lever to affect alignment in an exotrope are highly desirable. Absence of anisometropia is also a favorable indicator. In an esotrope, the presence of normal retinal correspondence on all tests is a positive sign. Presence of ARC on any tests would tend to reduce the probabilities of a functional outcome but would not necessarily preclude success. In exotropia, anomalous retinal correspondence on certain tests can be ignored if the strabismus is intermittent. Many intermittent exotropias of the divergence excess type will show ARC when in deviated posture and normal retinal correspondence when aligned. From a practical standpoint this demonstration of ARC may be ignored, for as alignment is achieved the retinal correspondence takes care of itself through covariation. Constant exotropia, particularly if it is basic with large deviation at both distance and near, is usually more productively managed if the patients are likened to esotropes in determining prognosis. Intermittent exotropia has exceedingly high functional cure rate with orthoptics. The same cannot be said with certainty of constant basic exotropia. Demonstration of fusional capability, particularly fusional vergence capacity, is an excellent prognostic sign. In general, patients with fusional vergence, normal retinal correspondence, intact motor systems, and no optical problems should achieve functional cure. Depending on the angle of turn the cure may be effected with orthoptics alone, or in combination with surgery. In certain instances, surgery by itself may produce functional results.

Another important factor is the anticipated change in function in the normal environment. If daily function is better when the patient is binocular than when the patient is not, one can reasonably expect that treatment will proceed more efficiently. This is so because of heightened patient motivation and also by virtue of reinforcing effects of daily activity. The converse also exists. This author has encountered esotropic patients who had been responding quite well to orthoptics until such time as they began to develop a heavy interest in reading. At that particular stage in treatment they were ineffectively and uncomfortably binocular. Since they could not function in a standard environment as binocular persons, they reverted to suppression and the turn angle increased. The heavy near point accommodative demands and the discomfort produced by fragile and unstable fusion was more disturbing than reverting to strabismus with deeper suppression. In many instances this situation is predictable and a change in the timing of therapy and possible convex lens prescription should be considered.

Planning the management of a strabismic problem must also include consideration of risk-benefit as well as cost-benefit factors. The former include the previously discussed possibility of the patient actually being worse after treatment than before. It is pointless to eliminate suppression unless there is the possibility of achieving alignment. It is unfair to offer surgery where there is high probability of diplopia or consecutive strabismus; anesthesia and health risks attendant to surgery must also be considered (Burian and von Noorden, 1980). Cost-benefit factors must be weighed not only in terms of money but of time and discomfort. The relationship between tangible benefits and the rigors of treatment must be considered. Persistent attempts to maintain acuity in an amblyopic eye in the absence of fusion may require almost constant therapy, which in itself reduces the patient's ability to function effectively.

It is essential that the decision include consideration of anticipated long-term consequences both without and with treatment. The question must be asked as to anticipated outcome if the condition is left untreated or if treatment is delayed until a later date. Frequently, parents are frightened into accepting surgery for strabismus for purposes of arresting or curing amblyopia before a child reaches age six or seven. This is not warranted for several reasons. Unless there is restoration of bifoveal fixation with full binocular function, the patient still has to suppress the fovea of the deviating eye. In most instances, amblyopia does not respond directly to surgical intervention. Furthermore, while there is good reason to institute amblyopia treatment procedures, such as refractive correction and stimulation of a turned eye, at as early an age as is possible, this does not mean that amblyopia cannot be treated at later dates. The age at which amblyopia develops is a more important factor in prognosis than the age at which active therapy is begun, particularly after the first few years of life. It may be more prudent to wait until the child is sufficiently mature, to assure more effective diagnosis and cooperation. Amblyopia treatment begun after age six is no less effective than that begun before this age (Birnbaum et al., 1977; Flom, 1970).

The anticipated results of treatment must be evaluated not only for their immediate impact but also for the long-term effects. Surgery for a strabismus is generally contraindicated when there is a strong accommodative component in the form of hyperopia that will almost certainly have to be corrected later in life. As long-term consequences are evaluated, it becomes apparent that compromise therapies may often be desirable. Given a poor prognosis for functional success, cosmetic surgery is certainly warranted. Partial functional results may also be a realistic objective of treatment. So long as the end result is cosmetically satisfactory and functionally useful it is sometimes appropriate to aim for peripheral fusion with stereopsis, leaving residual amblyopia and lack of bifoveal binocular function. Converting a large-angle turn to a stable and functionally useful mini-squint is not a failure but rather a resounding success from the patient's point of view. Naturally, it would be desirable to achieve full bifoveal alignment, full acuity, and central stereopsis but this is not always a practical goal. Similarly, there are instances in which control rather than cure should be the immediate objective. In the case of amblyopia where binocularity cannot be achieved, it is useful to improve the acuity of the amblyopic eye with intensive patching, pleoptics, and orthoptics just to establish a base-line capability in that eye. This has the very practical advantage of ensuring against blindness in case of injury to the normal eye and provides an enormous psychological benefit to the patient who no longer has one "blind eye." Then it might be well to permit the acuity to fall in that eye with occasional treatment to perk up the acuity rather than attempting constantly to maintain acuity against an impossible circumstance. Acuity will not be maintained unless full functional binocularity is achieved or the patient is made to alternate. Not all patients, for a variety of reasons, can become alternators.

Finally, it is important that strabismus be considered a disorder of a person. While some of the factors to be considered in diagnosis and prognosis reside in the eyes or the oculomotor system, the most important consideration should be the responses and behaviors of a person rather than of a pair of eyes. A humanistic assessment of the behaviors and problems of strabismus is required to provide maximal benefit. The therapeutic thrust should be to permit each and every patient to achieve the greatest improvement in ocular and overall performance as a consequence of appropriate diagnosis and management of the strabismus condition.

References

Amigo G, Fiorentini A, Pirchio M, Spinelli D. Binocular vision tested with visually evoked potentials. Invest Ophthalmol 1978 17(9):910-15.

Atkinson J, Braddick O, French J. Infant astigmatism: its disappearance with age. Vis Res 1980;20:891-93.

Ballen PH. Surgical treatment of intermittent exotropia. J Pediatr Ophthalmol 1970;7:55.

Birnbaum MH, Koslowe K, Sanet R. Success in amblyopia therapy as a function of age: a literature survey. Am J Optom 1979;54(5):269-75.

Blakemore C. Maturation and modification in the developing visual system. In: Held R, Liebowitz MW, Tauber ML, eds. Handbook of Sensory Physiology. Vol.8. Springer-Verlag, 1974:Berlin, New York: 377-436.

Blakemore C. The conditions required for the maintenance of binocularity in the kitten's visual cortex. J Physiol 1976;261:423-44.

Brock F. Binocular vision in strabismus. Optom Wkly 1945;36(3):67-8;179-80.

Brock F. Visual training. Part III. Optom Weekly 1956;2011-148.

Burian HM. Fusional movements in permanent strabismus. A study of the rule of central and peripheral retinal regions in the act of binocular vision in squint. Arch Ophthalmol 1941;26:626.

Burian HM. Sensorial retinal relationship in concomitant strabismus. Trans Am Ophthalmol Soc 1945;81:373.

Burian HM. Anomalous retinal correspondence, its essence and its significance in prognosis and treatment. Am J Ophthalmol 1951;34:237-53.

Burian HM. Occlusion amblyopia and the development of eccentric fixation in occluded eyes. Am J Ophthalmol 1966;62:853.

Burian HM, Spivey BE. The surgical management of exodeviations. Am J Ophthalmol 1965;59:603.

Burian HM, von Noorden GK. Binocular vision ocular motility, theory and management of strabismus. 2nd ed. St. Louis: CV Mosby, 1980.

Cooper J. Intermittent exotropia of the divergence excess type. J Am Opt Assoc 1977;48(10):1261-73.

Cooper J, Feldman J. Operant conditioning and assessment of stereopsis in young children. Am J Optom 1978a;55(8):532-44.

Cooper I, Feldman J. Random-dot-stereogram performance by strabismic, amblyopic, and ocular-pathology patients in an operant discrimination task. Am J Optom 1978b;55(9):599-609.

Cooper J, Feldman J. Panoramic viewing, visual acuity of deviating eye, and anomalous retinal correspondence in the intermittent exotrope of the divergence excess type. Am J Optom 1979;56(7):422-29.

Duckman R. The incidence of visual anomalies in a population of cerebral palsied children. J Am Opt Assoc 1979;50(9):1013-16.

Flax N. The optometric treatment of intermittent divergent strabismus. Eastern Seaboard Vision Training Conference, Washington, D, January, 1963.

Flax N. Training intermittent exotropes. San Jose Vision Training Seminar, August, 1968.

Flax N. Problems in relating visual function to reading disorder. Am J Optom 1970;47(5):369-70.

Flax N, Duckman R. Orthoptic treatment of strabismus. J Am Opt Assoc 1978;49(9):1353-61.

Flom MC. A minimum strabismus examination. J Am Opt Assoc 1956;27(11):643.

Flom MC. Treatment of binocular anomalies of vision, in Vision of Children. In: Hirsch MJ, Wick RE, eds. Philadelphia: Chilton Book Co., 1963:197-211.

Flom MC. Early experience in the development of visual coordination. In: Young FA, Lindsley DB, eds. Early experience and visual information processing in perceptual and reading disorders. Washington, D.C., National Academy of Sciences, 1970:291-99.

Flom MC. Corresponding and disparate retinal points in normal and anomolous correspondence. Am J Optom 1980;57(9):656-65.

Goldrich SG. Optometric therapy of divergence excess strabismus. Am J Optom 1980;57(1):7-14.

Goldrich SC. Oculomotor biofeedback therapy for exotropia. Am J Optom 1982;59(4):306-17.

Graham PA. Epidemiology of strabismus. Br J Ophthalmol 1974;58(3):224-31.

Griffin JR. Binocular anomalies-procedures for vision therapy. Chicago: Professional Press, 1976.

Griffin JR, Boyer FM. Strabismus measurement with the Hirschberg test. Opt Weekly 1974;65(32):34.

Hallden U. Fusional phenomena in anomalous correspondence. Acta Ophthalmol 1952;37:(Suppl)1-93.

Harcourt B. Strabismus affecting children with multiple handicaps. Br J Ophthalmol 1974;58:272-80.

Hardesty HH, Boynton JR, Keenan JP. Treatment of intermittent exotropia. Arch Ophthalmol 1978;96:268.

Hiles DA. Galket RJ. Plaster cast arm restraints and amblyopia therapy. J Pediatr Ophthalmol 1974;11(3):151-52.

Hirons R, Yolton RL. Biofeedback treatment of strabismus: case studies. J Am Opt Assoc 1978;49(8):875-82.

Hubel DH, Wiesel T. Binocular interaction in striate cortex of kittens reared with artificial squint. J Neurophysiol 1965:28:1041-59.

Hugonnier R, Hugonnier SC. Strabismus. heterophoria, ocular motor paralysis. Troutman SV, trans. St. Louis: CV Mosby, 1969.

Ikeda H, Wright MJ. A possible neurophysiological basis for amblyopia. Br Orthopt J 1975;32:2013.

Jones R, Eskridge JB. The Hirschberg test-a re-evaluation. Am J Optom 1970;47(2):105-44.

Kerr K. Vergence-induced correspondence changes in anomalous retinal correspondence. University microfilms, Ann Arbor, Mich., 1969.

Kerr K. Accommodative and fusional vergence in anomalous correspondence. Am J Optom 1980;57(9):676-80.

Lang J. Evaluation in small angle strabismus or microtropia. Arruga M, ed. International Strabismus Symposium. Basel, New York: S. Karger, 1968:219.

Ludlam WM. Strabismus definition. In: Borish IM, ed. Clinical refraction. 3rd ed. Chicago: Professional Press, 1970.

Maddox EE. The clinical use of prisms and the decentering of lenses. 2nd ed. Bristol, England: John Wright & Sons, 1893.

McLaughlin SC. Visual perception in strabismus and amblyopia. Psych Monogr General and Applied 1964; 78(12):1-23.

Mitchell DE, Freeman RD, Millodot M, Haegerstrom G. Meridional amblyopia: evidence for modification of the human visual system by early visual experience. Vision Res 1973;13:535-58.

Mohindra I, Held R, Gwiazda J, Brill S. Astigmatism in infants. Science 1978;202:329-31.

Morgan MW. Anomalous correspondence interpreted as a motor phenomenon. Am J Optom 1961;38(3):131-48.

Morgan MW. Anomalies of binocular vision. In: Hirsch MJ, Wick RE, eds. Vision of children. Philadelphia: Chilton Book Co., 1963:178-79.

Morgan MW. The Maddox classification of vergence eye movements. Am J Optom 1980;57(9):537-39.

Movshon JA, Chambers BEI, Blakemore C. Stereopsis and interocular transfer. Perception 1972;1:483-Y0.

Parks MM. Second thoughts about the pathophysiology of monofixational phoria. Am Orthoptic J 1964;14:159

Parks MM. The monofixational syndrome. Trans Am Ophthalmol Soc 1969;67:609.

Pratt-Johnson JA, Barlow JM, Tilson G. Early surgery for intermittent exotropia. Am J Ophthalmol 1977;84:689.

Raab EL, Parks MM. Recession of the lateral recti. Arch Ohthalmol 1969;82:203.

Reinecke RD, Simons K. A new stereoscopic test for amblyopia screening. Am J Ophthalmol 1974;78(4):714-21

Revell MJ. Strabismus, a history of orthoptic techniques. London: Barrie & Jenkins, 1971:1-6.

Richards W. Stereopsis and stereoblindness. Exp Brain Res 1969;10:380-88.

Roberts J. Eye examination findings among children. Vital Health Statistics 1972;11:115.

Roberts J. Eye examination findings among youth 12-17 years. Vital Health Statistics 1975;11:155.

Ronne G, Rindziunski E. The pathogenesis of anomalous correspondence. Acta Ophthalmol 1953;31:347.

Rosenberg R, Flax N, Brodsky R, Ahelman S. Accommodative levels under conditions of asymmetric convergence. Am J Optom 1953;30(5):244-54.

Spache GD. Investigating the issues of reading disability. Boston: Allyn & Bacon, 1976;47.

Thomas J, Mohindra I, Held R. Strabismic amblyopia in infants. Am J Optom 1979;56(3):197-201.

Van Sluyters RC. Recovery from monocular stimulus deprivation amblyopia in the kitten. Ophthalmology 1978; 85:478-88.

Windsor CE. Surgery, fusion, and accommodative convergence in exotropia. J Pediatr Ophthalmol 1971;8:166.

Worth C. Squint-its causes, pathology and treatment. Philadelphia: C Blakiston's Son, 1921.

STRABISMUS MANAGEMENT

Even before completing my optometry program at Columbia, I had decided that vision training was the field I wanted to be in. After approximately a year and a half of general practice, I stopped dispensing and limited the practice to training. Initially, the specialty practice was heavy with strabismus cases referred from optometric colleagues.

I had a fairly solid background in what I refer to as "British" orthoptics. This approach, is well presented in texts such as Practical Orthoptics by Lyle and Jackson (Blackiston, 1941) and The practice of Orthoptics by Giles (Hammond, Hammond & Co. 1943). Treatment utilizes closed instrument and central targets, in a direct frontal attack beginning at the angle of turn. The patient is taken through first, second, and third degree targets (simultaneous perception of dissimilar targets, flat fusion, and stereopsis targets in that order.) Anomalous retinal correspondence is dealt with head on in the amblyoscope with the instrument set at the objective angle. With a simultaneous target (such as a dog before one eye and a dog house before the other), the patient with ARC initially sees a dog outside of the house. By utilizing flashing, movement of the targets, and strong suggestion, the patient is brought to a stage of "binocular triplopia", seeing a dog outside the house and another in the house at the same time. Gradually, the patient is encouraged to fade the "wrong" dog and to see the correctly projected dog inside the house. Once NRC is established and suppression eliminated, fusion range is developed to achieve alignment

This treatment is brutal in its intensity on both patient and doctor. While not always successful, it often works. I have often thought that every optometrist should be made to experience "breaking" ARC in an amblyoscope at least one time. Certainly those actively engaged in strabismus therapy should be familiar with this method. Just one instance of a patient experiencing binocular triplopia forever changes one's thinking about ARC. At the very least, it makes one question the terminology that has been adopted by convention. The one place that could not be the locus of the anomaly is the retina. In earlier days the term utilized was "anomalous projection," a far better description of the phenomenon.

I also was familiar with the work of Fred Brock, a unique clinician-scientist who set up deceptively simple devices and experiments in his office. These were published over a number of years, primarily in the Optometric Weekly, more than a half century ago. The Optometric Weekly articles are not readily available and are not in the current "style" for scientific papers. Brock did small experiments on few patients and made little use of statistical analysis, but his insights and theoretical analysis were powerful. Sadly, while many of Brock's contributions to optometry and vision care are still being utilized, younger practitioners hardly recognize the name and many older ones have little understanding of his thinking. Optometrists use the Brock string, BU stereoscope cards, BSM anaglyphs, and other training techniques he invented with little appreciation of his underlying philosophy and how it evolved over many years of treating strabismus.

Fred Brock had a long career, during which his understanding and approach to strabismus evolved. Beginning with the traditional orthoptic approach, his clinical work and research led him to pioneer a very different approach to treatment. In a 1966 article (A Chronicle of Orthoptic History Covering 25 Years of Practice, The Optometric Weekly, Feb. 1966) he described a number of ingenious methods of establishing retinal rivalry, then normal foveal correspondence using dissimilar targets placed on the line of sight of each eye, followed by development of physiological diplopia, and then diplopia–to-fusion training. He noticed that some patients did not fuse images before each eye, but rather "reported seeing twin objects sliding through each other or climbing around each other," a condition called "Horror Fusionis." He stated: "We found that many subjects who had shown 3-D ability on the Brock Rings (at close range) later exhibited fusion aversion ... .This gave impetus to the idea that orthoptic training should proceed from the periphery inward." To my knowledge, this was the beginning of optometric emphasis on peripheral training, something which has had profound influence on all aspects of vision therapy.

Few people have had as profound an impact on an area of clinical activity as had Fred Brock. A lifetime of imaginative and creative clinical and investigative work has led to a strabismus management approach which, despite its enormous success, thus far has yet to be fully tapped.

The third major influence on my approach to treating strabismus was A.M. Skeffington. The OEP model offered a possible explanation for etiology of various types of strabismus. The treatment regimen that I developed for divergent excess strabismus is a synthesis of concepts I derived from Brock and Skeffington. More important for me was the over-arching concept that all visual adaptations were but part of a total organism response. Actually, it was through my work with strabismic patients that I came to more fully appreciate the "four circle" model, particularly what Skeffington labeled the speech-auditory component. Many esotropes, particularly those of early onset, do not possess the concepts necessary to be able to appreciate stereopsis. They reject "seeing" what they do not understand. Successful treatment of strabismus involves making it possible for the patient to develop the appropriate logic and language structures necessary to properly synthesize and utilize binocular inputs.

A phenomenon often noted when training strabismic patients is a reduction of the turn angle early in the treatment program even before any binocular procedures have been introduced. Historically, traditional orthoptics had no place for monocular training procedures other than those directed at acuity improvement for an amblyopic eye. Patients with convergence insufficiency, for instance, were treated to develop fusion and extend convergence ranges. No attention was paid to development of monocular skills. The influence of monocular procedures on the angle of turn are not accounted for in traditional orthoptics but make sense in the Skeffington model.

Two papers follow. The first, although never published, was presented in 1980 at a symposium on Fred Brock's work held at the American Academy of Optometry. The second, written in 1963, discusses the application of the Skeffington model to treatment of binocular problems.

BROCK'S TECHNIQUES

**Nathan Flax, O.D.
Presented at a symposium titled:
Perspectives on the contribution of Frederick Brock
American Academy of Optometry , 1980, unpublished**

Fred Brock had a career-long interest in strabismus. Over a span of more than 30 years, he theorized, investigated, and published prolifically. From the onset, he was deeply interested in the problem of retinal correspondence, and devoted considerable effort to understanding and explaining binocular vision in strabismus. His research generally utilized only a few observers and very simple devices, yet his insightful analysis led to major theoretical and practical clinical innovations.

A number of basic principles evolved and guided Brock's management of strabismus. These may be listed as follows:

1) Stereoscopic awareness includes all extrinsic objects from infinity to within a few inches of the eyes. Objects are perceived as single even if they are not within Panum's areas. (Brock contrasted this to the "true fusion" range limited by Panum's areas.)

2) The awareness of physiological diplopia is an entirely abnormal experience.

3) A final process of elaboration (beyond that of "true fusion") must be postulated to account for the existing isomorphism between actual and perceived space.

4) In normal binocular vision, retinal correspondence affords a plane of reference for spatial judgments. In strabismus, the patient utilizes other spatial cues to determine if the image in each eye belongs to a single object in space.

5) The adapted squinter retains a more factual awareness of the existing test situation than does the non-squinter. (i.e., The adapted squinter perceives the Brock single string as it actually is. He/she does not experience physiological diplopia wherein neither of the perceived strings is located where the real string actually is.)

6) Diplopia in habitual seeing represents a deterioration in visual function.

7) The alternator represents a further departure from normal than does the monolateral strabismic. Since he felt that the alternator was far more apt to develop ARC than the monolateral strabismic, Brock viewed ARC as more difficult to treat than was monocular suppression.

8) Stereopsis is more fundamental than simultaneous perception or flat fusion.

Early in Brock's career, he utilized the then standard techniques for development of physiological diplopia, retinal rivalry, and training at the objective angle in the amblyoscope to make the anomalously corresponding patient aware of binocular triplopia. He soon began to develop new approaches. In 1941, he wrote of the use of logic and reasoning in treatment of ARC. He used explanations and demonstrations to the patient to make them aware that they saw differently from normals.

Other techniques that he utilized were diplopia awareness on a very small light bulb held very close to the eye within the centration range, lustre through closed lid, projection training using a ring light held close to one eye which was projected around another target seen by the other eye, peripheral stereo on stationery ring targets at the centration point, and also a device known as the arrow-disc trainer. This latter device utilized prism to align targets with arrows on the line of sight of each eye to act as markers for each line of sight. One of the objectives stated by Brock in 1941 was that factual awareness (anomalous projection) must be changed to visual falsification (normal projection). Brock was referring to the fact that the anomalously projecting individual tended to report veridically and was unaware of normal physiological diplopia (which Brock labeled visual falsification since the percept does not coincide with the factual stimulus.)

Brock felt that fusion training should begin in periphery and gradually include center. Fusion targets at the outset were to be large, easily fused, possess a low visual acuity demand, and not have central fusible targets.

Brock also believed very strongly in utilization of logic and reasoning to condition squinters to normal habits prior to what he called muscle training. Brock felt that "when a patient lacked stereopsis, he does not speak the same language as we do." To this end he attempted to supply the patient with a logical structure to permit normal retinal projection.

Over the years there was a gradual change in Brock's approach. Physiologic diplopia training tended to be eliminated with emphasis shifting to work at the centration point and cultivation of peripheral stereopsis. Brock felt that it was not diplopia, but a demand for high performance that improved convergence performance on stick-in-straw test.

By 1957, Brock's philosophy had changed significantly and he stated "Most present day training methods are directed toward elimination of ARC and suppression by going through flat fusion, color lustre, and retinal rivalry, eventually leading to stereopsis. But if 3-D responses can be elicited at the outset along with bifixation, then this is the preferred method of starting squint training." He proposed therefore that training be done at close distances within the centration point and he further felt that amblyopia was not a deterrent to binocular organization provided that there is a binocular centration ability.

Early in 1959, Brock became increasingly concerned about posture as a significant aspect of binocular fixation. He felt that postural set and anticipation were important for bifixation. Later that year, Brock commented on then standard strabismus training approaches. He felt that early correction of refractive error was good. His feelings on amblyopia were somewhat at variance with standard philosophy. He felt that while occlusion therapy is good for the amblyopia, it tended to force alternation and this he felt was not desirable since the alternator adapts in a manner further from normal than does a unilateral strabismus. He proposed utilization of half-occluders to serve as a stopgap method to prevent alternation type adaptation. In general, when Brock referred to alternation type adaptation, he was referring to anomalous correspondence. He felt that establishment of normal retinal correspondence was of prime importance and he questioned the necessity to eliminate low acuity in the squinting eye to achieve this.

Brock also questioned the emphasis on development of simultaneous awareness of non-fusible targets (first degree fusion). He felt that this might be useful if mental effort were incorporated to bring the objects closer together but other than this he felt no strong need for this type of therapy. He further felt that antisuppression training was useless in cases of anomalous retinal correspondence since there was no need for diplopia in the presence of ARC.

Brock felt that the bifoveal stimulation in amblyoscope which was then prevalent could work, but he proposed alternative strategies for the management of strabismus. He proposed that treatment begin with closed lid lustre, and then proceed to color lustre utilizing targets such as the BU-l and 2 cards and then he recommended that a "projection box" be used whereby one eye viewed a ring of light held very, very close to the eye while the other eye fixated a distant target. The objective was then to move the ring light further and further from the patient while retaining the visual alignment of the two targets. Brock commented on diplopia awareness training indicating that this assumes that a fusion reflex will then spontaneously operate. He felt that this was not necessarily so and that a fusion reflex was not always present and could even be lost in cases where it had been present previously.

At the same time, Brock offered new directions in training, advocating investigation and measurement of the centration. range, and setting up of training procedures which demanded binocularity for successful completion. He also suggested working with younger children. His major thrust was the extension of the range of bifixation to the eventual elimination of squint without creating spatial distortion (diplopia) in anticipation of future gains. This seemed to be the culmination of his earlier work. The notion of diplopia training was abhorrent to Brock and he proposed a method of developing alignment in strabismus without going through what he felt to be the unnecessary and artificial circumstance of creating diplopia.

The method proposed to do this was based upon the utilization of the stereo-motivator and BSM Series. The intent was to induce binocular performance without awareness of diplopia. Characteristically, this training began at near and proceeded to further distances; it began peripherally and proceeded to more central targets. Important in the training approach was cultivation of SILO responses and spatial localization as well as singleness and stereopsis. Part of the treatment procedure involved the attempt on the patient to manually manipulate virtual objects. This objective could be met utilizing anaglyphs as in the BSM Series and also by use of vectographic material.

Another important aspect of this training approach was the development of procedures to create a demand for binocular participation. Among procedures utilized for this purpose were the pointer in tube technique whereby a patient was asked to make a critical distance localization judgment at near and also the use of what Brock called "multiple pointers" which involved the manipulation of a virtual image to be placed on real targets.

Brock felt that surgery should be utilized if it was not possible to find a centration point for the start of this type of training with the use of either lenses and/or prisms. Failing this, he felt that surgery had to be utilized to give a beginning point for ultimate development.

Brock was keenly aware of the overall organismic aspects of his patient and appreciated the fact that the strabismic adaptation characteristically was made in the interests of preserving viability of performance. One of his admonitions was to avoid training circumstances which might force the strabismic into a disadvantageous adaptation. Even though the squinter had difficulty communicating with the non-squinter because of a different utilization of the various cues available for spatial judgments, nonetheless the squinter did possess a method of functioning in the world. This was not to be rudely disrupted. He was concerned that overzealous treatment to overcome suppression or to normalize retinal correspondence might cause the patient to develop diplopia or confusion which he felt to be a less effective status. The use of peripheral stereopsis and training of fusion at a finite centration point served to reinforce normal performance, whereas training, at the objective angle with emphasis on diplopia awareness would carry higher risk of causing a disadvantageous adaptation.

Toward the latter stages of Brock's career, he devised techniques which placed greater emphasis on home activity and he became more concerned about the role of posture and preset or anticipation in maintaining alignment. It was during this period that he developed the "posture board" based upon the notion of providing feedback cues to the patient regarding eye posture as well as traditional fusional cues.

Throughout Brock's career, he showed keen appreciation and understanding of the strabismic individual as a person with a need to compensate and cope. This underlying consideration of the totality of the patient's behavior was present at all times. He felt that inasmuch as the purpose of all sensory perception is to act, it was necessary to consider the effect of the lowered efficiency of an individual on his performance capacity when making any therapeutic decision. This type of thinking was perhaps fundamental to his apparent lack of concern about amblyopia in favor of concern about binocular integration. Characteristically, the amblyopia per se does not have as significant an impact on the performance of the squinter in a normal world (with neither eye occluded) as does the turn itself.

Brock keenly appreciated the fact that anomalously projecting strabismics (ARC), in particular, show rather remarkably satisfactory ability to make real judgments in a real world. Because of this Brock was concerned about the possibility of creating worse problems by solving lesser ones and he even questioned the justification in interfering with the fully adapted anomalous corresponding strabismic.

Much of what Brock offered is now considered relatively standard therapy although by no means is it universally applied. This is unfortunate since the strabismus management techniques developed by Fred Brock have enormous potential for effective treatment of strabismus and yet carry with them little or no downside risk of leaving patient worse after treatment than before.

This is an inherent problem in management of strabismus, often occurring after surgery. There is also risk present in some strabismus techniques which are primarily directed toward establishment of diplopia awareness in the hope that a fusion reflex will then spontaneously resolve the problem. This is not always the case. Brock's techniques can succeed where the others fail and does so in a manner minimally disruptive to the function of the patient.

New Concepts on the Control of Binocular Deviations

Nathan Flax, O.D.
J Am Opt Assoc 1963;34(60):451-5

Consultant, Optometric Center of New York;
Member AOA Committee on Visual Problems of Children and Youth.
Presented at Symposium on Binocular Imbalance, October 21, 1962, New York, New York.

Recent years have seen a change in the optometric concept of vision. Whereas the traditional approach had emphasized optical considerations, there is now greater interest in the perceptual aspects of the process of vision. More and more, the working hypothesis upon which clinical care is based has moved from a camera analogy of vision to that of a data processing system. As attempts have been made to explore the mechanisms whereby the data of sight are converted into meaningful constructs, understanding of the elements of visual perception has broadened considerably. Borrowing from our colleagues in physiology, psychology, education, engineering, and mathematics, we in optometry have revised our thinking concerning the role of the various ocular mechanisms.

Reappraisal of the Optical System

Vision is now considered as an information gathering sense modality, with the perceptual and cognitive aspects an integral part of the total process. The roles of the various ocular mechanisms are being reevaluated with this in mind. The newer understanding compels closer scrutiny of the means by which the organism obtains useful information from light energy. This search for a more useful working model for vision is proceeding along several major lines. One avenue of approach concerns itself with reappraisal of the optical system of the eye itself.

The "emmetropic perfect" eye demonstrates itself as being somewhat sterile in its ability to serve as an optimum link in the chain for transmitting the perceptual content of light energy. The "refractive error" is now seen to have utility as a perceptual mechanism since the visual system seems to have the ability to monitor itself and to gain awareness from the very act of maintaining focal adjustment. In the developing visual system, the optics of the eye seem to correspond to various stages of the learning of spatial relationships and, indeed, some astigmatic as well as hyperopic and myopic refractive states seem to relate to the individual's ability and need to adjust his ocular mechanisms to permit a more useful structuring of visual-perceptual spatial relationships.

In the same vein, the optical distortions of the eye may serve perceptual purposes. Chromatic aberration, for instance, seems vital to the proper control of accommodation. This mechanism adjusts in the proper direction in white light but operates randomly in monochromatic light. This would certainly imply that useful information is being obtained from the "aberration", which would seem undesirable on a purely optical basis.

This utilization of the data provided by the "imperfection" is in keeping with the newer visual model whereby vision operates as a regulatory mechanism with feed-back control, sensing its own oscillations and responding to them. The key point here is the fact that if there were no errors, and consequently no oscillations, there would be no data and no perceptual awareness despite a perfect optical system.

This same concept is applicable to the extrinsic muscle aiming system of the eyes. The visual system apparently monitors the adjusting movements and derives valuable information from the motor movements themselves. In the matter of visual form perception, for instance, there would seem to be a direct relationship between the ability (at a particular stage in visual development) to move eyes around a contour and the ability to recognize the shape of the contour. This awareness of the role of extra-ocular muscle proprioception as part of the total perceptual process in vision has enormous implications in the area of binocular imbalance and strabismus. Successful management of strabismus must take this factor into account.

Role of the Motor System
Some aspects of this are being widely considered. The role of the motor system in the matter of normal and anomalous projection has been most analytically stated by Morgan. The pleoptic techniques now in vogue involve a great deal of matching of ocular direction with kinesthesia of hand and arm. Interestingly, the new pleoptic techniques bear striking resemblance to many older optometric visual training procedures.

The motor aspects of binocular control and visual perception can only be fully appreciated in the context of vision as a partially innate, but largely acquired skill. The newer concepts of binocular control require understanding of how the perceptual values of motor movements are established and how the individual utilizes this information to fulfill the role of vision. This role is the acquiring of information from light We must go beyond the purely ocular mechanisms themselves for this understanding. The structuring of visual data requires a datum or baseline for meaningful organization and such a baseline could not derive from eyes alone. To be useful, the spatial construct of vision must match the spatial constructs of all of the other sensory-motor systems of the body. Perceived visual space must match perceived auditory and kinesthetic space. The perceived visual space must be consistent with the previous experience of the individual in order to be fully useful as a source of information. Visual perceptions must relate to the verbal constructs of the individual in order to become fully integrated and meaningful.

Integration with Other Motor Systems
The new concept of control of binocular deviation aims for much more than eyes which are straight and work one with the other in normal binocular fusion. The new concept sets the goal of straight eyes and a visual system capable of consistent integration with all of the other perceptuo-motor systems. Binocular control must extend beyond eyes and relate to over all bodily function.

The structuring of visual perception derives from bodily kinesthesia and, in particular, from posturing mechanisms. To a fairly large degree, vision is a balancing and steering mechanism. The value of paired eyes goes beyond the ability to appreciate stereopsis, for with two receptors, the human visual system is an excellent photo-postural mechanism. In this regard, it is worth noting that a significant portion of optic nerve fibers do not seem to enter the "seeing" portion of vision at all, but are intimately involved with the vestibular and postural mechanisms of the body.

This relationship of vision and gravity cannot be ignored in the management of binocular deviations. As a matter of fact, there is the possibility that the development of early binocular function is part and parcel of the development of a functional relationship between the two sides of the body in the process of learning to overcome gravity in locomotion. This would certainly seem to be so in the instances of reported strabismus "cures" among retarded children who have been taught to integrate the left and right sides of their bodies in crawling activities as part of motor therapy to teach them to walk.

There seems to be a growing awareness among many clinicians of a relationship between strabismus and distortions in the early childhood developmental sequence. It is interesting to note the frequency of reported omission of crawling or highly atypical crawling, for instance, among esotropic youngsters. This is not inconceivable in light of the concept of binocular function being a part of development of the working relationship of the two sides of the body.

Broadening the Base of Operation

These newer concepts in the control of binocular deviations in no way contradict any of the long accepted clinical tenets upon which optometric treatment has been based. They do not negate the value of standard treatment procedures. They do, however, broaden the base of operation and open new areas and techniques. They also offer better explanation for the results of some of the long accepted procedures.

In the light of consideration of the perceptuo-motor aspects of extra-ocular motor control, it is no wonder that surgery for strabismus produces such dismal results. A relationship between visual space and auditory, kinesthetic, and verbal space which has been developed over a period of years (even if the eyes are not parallel) cannot be rudely torn apart without enormous dislocations in perceptual matching. It is not surprising that so few post-operative patients ever manage to utilize their eyes as a team in normal binocular function, and still fewer ever become fully efficient at matching their visual systems to the rest of their bodily motor-perceptual systems. Many "cured" strabismics with straight eyes and some degree of fusion perform in their daily activities as if their eyes still turned.

It is also to be expected that orthoptically trained patients will show a greater degree of normal binocular function since there has been some opportunity for a gradual "reprogramming" of visual data so that perceptual integrity can be maintained. If this orthoptic training is confined to very circumscribed instrument procedures which restrict the field of view to the central retinal area, we can expect the therapy to have limited success. This is consistent with the fact that the peripheral retinal areas seem most related to postural activities and utilization of only central stimulation does not permit full realization of the goal of integration of visual cues with other cues of spatial orientation.

Peripheral Retinal Stimulation

Optometrically oriented visual training which involves considerable utilization of peripheral retinal stimulation and permits matching of kinesthetic and tactual data by training in "real space" as well as in instruments brings us closer to the goal of unification of sensory-motor systems of the entire body. This does not mean that instrument approaches are invalid or unwarranted. Indeed, there are many instances where the discrepancy between the existing modes of operation are so great as to make it impossible for the strabismic patient to bridge the gap without the use of the intervening transition stages possible only in the artificial environment of an optical instrument.

Monocular Training Procedures

This new understanding of vision gives insight into the value of monocular procedures in the treatment of binocular imbalance. Monocular pursuit and saccadic training have far greater utility than merely to teach central fixation and a normal eye-hand relationship in amblyopic patients. A carefully controlled monocular vision training routine can establish optimum conditions for binocular teaming by development of a match between spatial values of each eye with the other body systems before the two eyes are required to work together. Once the two eyes each develop a similar relationship with a common denominator outside the ocular system,. the process of matching the two ocular systems to one another is greatly simplified. It is much easier to train the relationship between visuomotor direction and bodily kinesthesia in a monocular training situation than in a binocular situation with a strabismic patient. A monocular training sequence which begins with tactual and proprioceptive cues to lead the eyes starts to develop the matching between visual information and bodily information. As the training situation is gradually modified so that the patient can respond properly to monocular visual data without need for kinesthetic reinforcement, the basis for easier integration of binocular visual data is established.

Involving Motor Bilateral Activities

The development of binocular integration can also be enhanced by incorporating training procedures which involve gross motor bilateral activities and also postural balancing mechanisms. Learning to walk erect involves a sequential series of motor activities which gradually lead to integration of the two body sides. Throughout this process, there is an interaction between balancing reflexes, vestibular control, and vision.

Just as binocular imbalances can lead to postural defects, so can postural disturbances influence ocular coordination. A matrix for proper binocular integration can be facilitated by utilization of visually controlled postural activities as part of a vision training sequence. Indeed, there are some instances where this type of activity seems to be the primary agent in effective elimination of strabismus.

Development of sound bi-manual control by utilization of chalkboard activities can aid the management of a binocular problem by providing a kinesthetic frame of reference for two-eyed performance. Integration of balancing procedures in a vision training program can assist in the restoration of normal binocular function by permitting integration of the postural data of sight with vestibular data and postural reflexes.

Concept of Unity of Perception

A most important aspect of the new approach to the management of binocular problems is the concept of the unity of perception by the various sense modalities and the recognition of the role of sensory-motor data in this perception. Insofar as possible, a vision training program must be programmed to conform with this concept. There must be opportunity for perceptuo-motor matching to take place in such a manner that visual data, or the visual perceptual world, can conform to the rest of the perceptions of the individual. This requires utilization of a multi-sensory approach. It also requires that the training program permit reinforcement by providing opportunity for all of the motor systems of the body to participate in addition to the ocular system itself.

References

1. Gesell A, Ilg FL, Bullis C. Vision, Its Development in Infant & Child. New York: Paul Hoeber, Inc., 1949.

2. *Getman GN. How to Develop Your Child's Intelligence. Santa Ana, CA: Optometric Extension Program, 2002. Originally published, Luverne, MN: by the author, 1962.*

3. *Harmon DB. Notes on a Dynamic Theory of Vision, 3rd Revision, vol. 1. Published by author, 1958.*

4. *Hebb DO. The Organization of Behavior. New York: John Wiley & Sons, Inc.,1949.*

5. *Kephart NC. The Slow Learner in the Classroom. Columbus, OH: Charles E. Merrill, 1960.*

6. *Ludlam WM. Orthoptic treatment of strabismus. Am J Optom 1961 Jul:369-388.*

7. *Morgan MW. Anomalous correspondence interpreted as a motor phenomenon. Am J Optom 1961 Mar:141-148.*

8. *Skeffington AM. Postgraduate Optometric Courses. Duncan, OK: Optometric Extension Program Foundation , 1926-1962.*

EFFECTIVENESS OF VISUAL THERAPY

Orthoptic treatment of strabismus is highly effective. Despite this, there have been problems in gaining recognition in insurance and governmental programs. It was difficulty with inclusion in such a program which prompted the writing of Orthoptic Treatment of Strabismus. Both the medical and optometric literature were reviewed. No attempt was made to select only favorable results. The papers were selected based upon just two criteria. The first was that the paper had to have a sufficiently clear statement of success criteria to permit analysis. The second criteria was that orthoptic training was the principle treatment used, rather than a combination of surgery and orthoptics. The available data showed impressive functional success rates in both the ophthalmological-orthoptist and optometric studies, although substantially better in the optometric studies. One wonders if the ophthalmologists read their own literature which showed a 56% functional cure rate by orthoptists (76% cure rate for optometrists). The paper also explains why optometric treatment is superior to training by orthoptic technicians and includes information on the training of optometrists.

The paper follows.

Orthoptic Treatment of Strabismus

Nathan Flax, O.D., M.S. and Robert H. Duckman, O.D., M.A.
J Am Optom Assoc 1978;49(12):1353-61

Abstract
The purpose of this paper will be to carefully examine the effectiveness of orthoptics as a viable treatment modality for strabismus. It will be necessary to first examine the scope of this problem and the significance of functional cure. A short discussion of perceptual and psychological effects will be included. A review of pertinent literature and an analysis of the data will be presented. Any commonalities or generalizations which can be identified will then be discussed and analyzed. Finally, the training of the optometrist in orthoptics and associated subjects will be examined to demonstrate the qualification of the optometrist to administer orthoptics in the treatment of visual anomalies.

Key Words
strabismus, fusion, tropia, heterotropia, squint, ocular deviation

Definition
Strabismus is the condition in which the two eyes are directed to different points when looking at an object in space. Under normal conditions, and in the absence of strabismus, the two eyes are directed to the same point when fixating an object. This deviating of one eye from the point of regard causes diplopia (double vision) and visual confusion which become the stimuli for suppression ("turning off" of visual input into the deviating eye). Tropia, heterotropia, squint, and manifest ocular deviation are other technical names for this condition. Terms such as "crossed eye" or "wall eye" are used in the popular vernacular.

Epidemiology

Graham[1] reports an incidence of manifest squint of approximately 5.5% of the total six-year-old population of the city of Cardiff. 4,784 children all born in one year were screened by an orthoptist and those with doubtful measurement on cover test were seen for a more detailed orthoptic evaluation. He also cites prior work by Frandsen who found a 6% incidence of manifest squint at age 6 years in Copenhagen.

According to surveys by the National Center for Health Statistics of the United States Department of Health, Education and Welfare,[2,3] the most common visual abnormality found in children ages 6 - 17 is strabismus. The incidence of strabismus in this age category is 6.72% or an estimated 1.6 million children. There are no apparent trends related to age or sex, but strabismus appears about twice as frequently in the Midwest as it does in any other area of the United States. Strabismus is also more prevalent among families where income is less than $5,000/year.

Psychological and perceptual considerations
There are two major factors involved in strabismus, both of which contribute to its disabling consequences. Usually, the most obvious aspect is the motor misalignment of the eyes. The appearance of the squint sufferer is often significantly altered from normal, resulting in obvious disfigurement

leading to such appellations as "cast in the eye" or "cockeyes." The effects of such a condition on personality development and interpersonal relationships can be enormous.

The second factor, although less obvious to the lay observer, can have even greater far reaching consequences. The human visual system is anatomically and physiologically arranged so that visual information is most appropriately assimilated when the two eyes team together and both aim at a common object of regard. Distance, size and directional judgments are dependent upon proper sensory integration data from the two eyes. The patient with strabismus suffers from disruption of the sensory processes of vision. In some instances, this sensory defect can result in double vision. In other cases, there is interference and error introduced in visual judgments which require two-eye coordination. Yet another consequence is the inhibition or suppression of vision of one eye, or amblyopia which can lead to loss of sight of an eye, sometimes irreversible.

Lipton[4] emphasizes the importance of considering effects of strabismus on a child's psychological development. He says:

The major thesis has been that strabismus may affect the individual as a unique form of trauma because of certain pathophysiological effects. These may be complicated by the reactions of the individual's environment to the nature of the defect. Of crucial importance is the child's distrust of his own perceptions and the resulting mental confusion. These factors interact with and influence the unfolding of the libidinal drives and aggression, the choice of defense mechanisms, and certain aspects of ego and superego development and functioning. Of great significance is the fact that strabismus usually has its onset at two and a half to five years-a period when the child is confronted by a great variety of developmental tasks.

Treatment objectives

While the cosmetically noticeable misalignment of the two eyes tends to attract attention to the problem more than the loss of eyesight and the functional disability caused by the sensory aspect of the condition, this latter facet requires treatment in order to normalize vision. Too often, the treatment of squint is directed entirely toward the cosmetic, totally ignoring functional considerations. Surgical treatment of strabismus produces complete functional binocular use of the eyes as a team in relatively few instances. It is not the purpose of this paper to argue the merits of strabismus surgery, but rather to present data on a treatment method, orthoptics, which can produce rather high *functional* cure rates-as well as cosmetic alignment of the eyes and improvement in eyesight. The desirability of restoration of visual acuity and normal physiological functioning of binocular vision is self-evident. Indeed, these should be the prime objectives of strabismus therapy.

Results of orthoptics in the treatment of strabismus

While orthoptics is not new, there is lack of agreement as to its efficiency. There are a number of reasons for this. Ludlam[5] reviewed 15 studies showing positive results ranging from 92.7% to 16%. He listed five basic faults in the papers, with each one suffering from one or more defects as follows:

A. Orthoptics was viewed as a secondary method of cure, to be used after surgery had not given the desired results. As a consequence, orthoptic and surgical results were reported so intertwined, that it was impossible to judge accurately the part played by orthoptics in the final results.

B. *No satisfactory specific and detailed definition of 'cure' or results was formulated, so that there could be no general agreement as to the results obtained in a specific case.*

C. *The training work unfortunately was performed largely, in the words of Law, by "medically unqualified certified orthoptists," who, quoting Douglas, "it must be remembered, have had only a minimum of scientific training."*

D. *Some of the quoted figures for rates of cure were rough estimates based on the recollection of the clinical experience of that author, and not based on a strict analysis or study. In several of the papers, too strict a selection policy in reporting cases has obscured the true value of orthoptics alone as a specific strabismus remedy for large numbers of strabismics.*

This paper will concern itself with a number of papers on the efficiency of orthoptics which largely avoid the basic faults listed by Ludlam. The papers included all have attempted orthoptics as a prime therapy and not secondary to surgery. They all present results which permit the isolation of orthoptic results from surgical procedures. Some have control groups. They state their success criteria with reasonable clarity, and have set a high functional standard for success.

Studies were located which indicate favorable results of orthoptics in the management of squint in both the ophthalmologic orthoptist and optometric literature. This distinction is made because there are differences in the orthoptic approaches, procedures, and strategies offered by the two groups, as well as in the education and preparation of the practitioners. This will be commented upon later in the paper.

Ophthalmological-orthoptist results

The ophthalmological-orthoptist studies[6-15] involve a total of 489 patients and report a total of 275 patients as successful functionally for a percentage cure of 56%. If an additional 17 cases who were straight with glasses (Zaki)[14] and 25 who were almost straight (Gillan)[9] are included, the success rate goes up to 67% (see Table #1). Combining papers in this way does not fully give the flavor of the results since the success criteria, patient samples, and orthoptic methods differ somewhat from study to study. The individual papers are summarized below:

Chryssanthou[6] reports on the orthoptic management of 27 cases of intermittent exotropia ranging in age from 5 to 33 years. 89% of the group showed definite improvement with 66.7% classified as excellent, 11.1% classified as good, and 11.1% classified as fair. The criteria for the various classifications are quite rigorous and well stated. Even in the second best "good" category, the requirements for success were:
 1) phoria for all distances
 2) absolute convergence ability greater than 20 prism diopters at distance and near
 3) a near point of convergence 5 centimeters or closer
 4) absence of suppression
 5) patient comfort without asthenopia
 6) fusion range in synoptophore from -3 degrees to +20 degrees

The criteria for the excellent category were even more demanding. It should be pointed out that these results were attained despite the fact that one-third of the sample had "appreciable hyperdeviations" and four had abnormal retinal correspondence. Both conditions tend to lower the possibilities of functional cure. Additionally, 55% of their sample were reported as having some degree of lateral gaze incomitance, another factor giving a poor prognosis. Chryssanthou states: "Considering the strict criteria used in our classification, the 89% of patients who showed improvement with 66.6% graded excellent or good, six months to 2-1/2 years after termination of the orthoptic treatment are impressive percentages."

San Filippo and Clahane[7] reported on 31 exotropes who were treated solely with orthoptics. They established rigorous criteria for success and used each patient in the investigation as its own control. They carefully assessed the binocular status both before and after treatment. Their criteria for evaluation of the binocular relationship were as follows:

Excellent:
1) Phoria for far distance, distance, and near in the primary position and reading position
2) Absolute convergence not less than 20 prism diopters for distance and near
3) Relative convergence not less than 15 prism diopters for distance and near
4) Unlimited near point of convergence
5) No suppression
6) Excellent awareness of diplopia during testing situation
7) Comfortable without asthenopic symptoms

Good:
1) Phoria for far distance, distance, and near in the primary and reading position
2) Absolute convergence not less than 15 prism diopters for distance and near
3) Relative convergence not less than 10 prism diopters for distance and near
4) Near point convergence 50mm. or closer
5) Slight central suppression
6) Good awareness of diplopia
7) Comfortable without asthenopic symptoms

Fair:
1) Intermittent at one testing distance only; phoria in the three remaining positions
2) Absolute convergence not less than 10 prism diopters for distance and near
3) Relative convergence not less than 5 prism diopters for distance and near
4) Near point convergence 70mm. or closer
5) Moderate peripheral and foveal suppression
6) Fair awareness of diplopia
7) Slight asthenopic symptoms; problems with diplopia

Poor:
1) Tropia at any distance or intermittent at two of the four testing distances
2) Absolute convergence less than 10 prism diopters for distance and near
3) Relative convergence less than 5 prism diopters for distance and near
4) Near point of convergence poorer than 80 mm
5) Peripheral and foveal suppression
6) No awareness of diplopia
7) Asthenopic symptoms

Each patient was used as his own control and was evaluated before and after the orthoptic treatment. Prior to therapy, 80.6% of the patients were poor and 19.4% were graded as fair. None were in the good or excellent category. Upon completion of treatment, 64.5% were graded as excellent, 9.7% graded as good, and 22.6% graded as fair. Only one patient still remained in the poor category. A long-term follow-up done 4- ½ to 6-1/2 years after orthoptic therapy showed 51.7% to still be in the excellent category and 16.1% in the good category. 68% of the patients were still in the good or excellent categories on this long-term evaluation of patients treated solely with orthoptics. 84% of the exotropes showed improvement over their initial status.

Altizer[8] reports on a comparison of 23 exotropes treated orthoptically with 29 treated surgically. While her success ratio with orthoptic treatment is somewhat less than reported by other authors, the orthoptically treated group still fared better than the surgically treated group. Ten of 23 orthoptically treated cases were considered to be controlled while only 11 of 29 surgically treated cases achieved that status. She concludes that surgical and non-surgical treatment of exotropia achieved fairly equal functional results.

Gillan[9] reports on 63 cases treated solely with orthoptics. Twenty-three became perfectly straight and 25 became almost straight. Only 15 of 63 orthoptically treated patients did not become almost straight or better. A control group was utilized using 50 cases who were on the waiting list for orthoptic treatment. These controls had only been treated with glasses. Not a single case in the control group showed a spontaneous cure and there was reduction of the squint angle in only 11 of the cases. The remainder were either stationary or had gotten worse. By contrast, 48 in the experimental group were made straight or almost straight. Their results show an incomparable superiority of results in the orthoptic group as against those treated only with glasses.

In a series of papers, Guibor[10-13] reported on a controlled experiment involving a series of orthoptically treated strabismics compared to a non-treated control group. The initial study included 38 orthoptically treated cases and 40 untreated cases. Experimental patients seen in Guibor's study all received intensive orthoptic treatment once weekly. The control group received refractive correction, occlusion, and atropinization where indicated. Both experimental and control groups were evaluated similarly for binocular fixation, binocular vision, and stereoscopic ability.

Of the orthoptic cases, 50% achieved alignment of the eyes with glasses, while another 34% showed improvement in the squint. Of the untreated control group who were treated with glasses, only 12.5% achieved alignment of the eyes, and only 25% showed any improvement in the squint. The contrast between the treated and untreated groups is striking. In the untreated control group, 62.5% of the patients showed no improvement in the squint, while among the orthoptically treated cases, only 16% showed no improvement. The modest improvement reported in the control group is undoubtedly due to the fact that they did receive some therapeutic attention that is included as part of an overall orthoptic program. But they did not receive specific binocular training procedures and the rather dramatic differences between the two groups is due to active orthoptic intervention. The orthoptically treated patients averaged five months of treatment with the longest cases requiring one year therapy. Guibor concluded that "there seemed to be no age limit in these cases beyond which it was impossible to develop fusion" and that "patients showing considerable amblyopia were capable of developing fusion in the stereoscope."

A follow-up study with additional cases demonstrated correction of the squint with glasses in 60% of the orthoptically treated cases. He reports: "Of the whole series, 50% could fuse accurately with the stereoscope, amblyoscope, and synoptophore with constant depth perception. An additional 40% had varying degrees of binocular perception."

Cooper and Leyman,[15] as part of a larger study, report on 182 intermittent exotropes treated solely with orthoptics. They report a 58.7% success rate with their good criteria defined as follows:
1) Phoria at 60 meters, 6 meters and 33 cm
2) Absolute convergence amplitude of 25 prism diopters at 6m and 35 prism diopters at 33 cm
3) Near point of convergence within 5 cm
4) Stereopsis at near of 40 seconds of arc
5) Fusion of Worth four dot at 6m
6) Appreciation of diplopia when dissociated
7) Good fusional recovery when dissociated

These results were better than those reported for a group of 264 treated with surgery alone (41.6%) and another group of 216 treated with combined orthoptics and surgery (52.3%). Cooper and Leyman point out that the orthoptic group tended to have smaller deviations than the operated group. Yet, comparison of the 55 patients in the orthoptics only group who had large deviations (25 prism diopters or more) with the operation only group shows that a higher percentage of combined good and fair results was obtained with orthoptics than with surgery.

They state: "In the United States, the distribution of orthoptists is such that not every ophthalmologist has one available, and of necessity he must confine his efforts to break down suppressing to the use of occlusion. Few ophthalmologists have time or inclination to do more but since orthoptic training obviously can benefit patients with intermittent exotropia, it seems reasonable that it should not be denied to them wherever facilities exist to provide it. It is our opinion that to confine the treatment of intermittent exodeviations to surgery only is to deny the patient a better chance for a good result."

Zaki[14] reports on orthoptics in the treatment of small angle deviations. One hundred twenty children five to seven years of age were selected on the basis of having a squint angle with correction of less than 12 degrees and no more than two lines difference between the corrected visual acuity of the two eyes. The patients were given intensive binocular training over a period of approximately 14 months. The success criteria established was fairly rigorous as follows:
1) The angle of deviation with +5 degrees to 0 with *and* without corrective lenses
2) Fusion on Worth four-dot test with *and* without lenses
3) Good stereopsis with *and* without lenses
4) The ability to bar read with *and* without lenses

Seventy-five of 120 cases achieved the cure criterion. Their best results were with accommodative and partially accommodative esotropias while they did not do as well with divergent strabismus. Even in this category, however, they achieved a 40% success rate. They achieved a 71.6% cure in partially accommodative esotropia. The fully accommodative esotropias achieved 100% success. The cure category required straight eyes *without* glasses This is an unusually stringent demand. Seventeen patients who were straight *with* glasses were called unsuccessful and were then operated on! Had these

TABLE 1
RESULTS OF OPHTHALMOLOGIC-ORTHOPTIST ORTHOPTICS

Study	Patients	Cosmetic & Functional Success	Functional Cure	Cosmetic Success	Overall Functional & Cosmetic Cure
Chryssanthau[6] (good or excellent both counted as functional result)	27	18	67%	-	67%
San Filippo and Clahane[7] (good and excellent counted as functional result)	31	23	74%	-	74%
Altizer[8]	23	10	43%	-	43%
Gillan[9]	63	23	37%	25	76%
Guibor[10-13]	38	19	50%	13	84%
Zaki[14] (Note: Others might have considered the 17 "cosmetic" cures as functional cures – see text)	125	75	60%	17	74%
Cooper and Lyman[15]	182	107	59%	-	59%
TOTALS	489	275	56%	55	67%

cases been considered successful (as most other strabismologists would have classified them) the cure rate would have been 74%.

Optometric results

The optometric[5,16,17,19,20] studies involve a total of 433 patients, 332 of whom achieved very high level functional cure results for a combined cure rate of 72.4% (see Table #2). If another 44 patients in the combined group whose eyes were straightened but who failed to meet the rigid functional criteria are included, the cure rate with optometric orthoptics becomes almost 87%! The individual papers are summarized below.

Layland[16] describes orthoptic techniques utilized at the London Refracting Hospital and reports that the deviation was eliminated in 14 of 15 cases of divergent squint. The criteria for cure required:
1) that there be recovery of the deviating eye after cover test in spite of a voluntary effort by the patient to maintain diplopia
2) the strabismus is not noted at any time by the patient or parent
3) the patient is symptom free
4) there is good voluntary convergence
5) there is no central suppression
6) fusion is present over the whole or all but the extreme upper part of the motor field
7) the patient has normal abductions and adductions

He also reports of another sample where 15 of 17 divergent squinters obtained good binocular vision after orthoptics. Nineteen others had no manifest deviation even though they did not pass all of the functional criteria. Combining the two samples, 72 of 107 cases achieved functional cure for a complete success rate of 67% while an additional 18% of the patients had straight eyes for an overall success of 85%.

Etting[17] reports on orthoptic training for 42 constant strabismics, ages 2 to 17 years. The criteria for case selection required that the strabismus be present at all distances with best refractive correction and that there be a minimum of 12 orthoptic treatments. The sample included 20 exotropes and 22 esotropes. The training period spanned from 12 to 94 orthoptic sessions. Seven of the patients had had surgery prior to orthoptics, 12 had anomalous correspondence, 14 had amblyopia, and 2 had eccentric fixation. An exceedingly rigorous success criteria was established based upon the prior work of Flom.[18] The success criteria required that:
1) there be clear, comfortable, single binocular vision at all distances up to the near point of convergence which itself had to be normal
2) there had to be stereopsis and normal ranges of motor fusion
3) occasional turning of the eye up to 1% of the time was permitted provided that the patient was aware of diplopia whenever it occurred
4) corrective lenses and small amounts of prism (up to 5 prism diopters) could be utilized

Sixty-four percent of this sample achieved a functional cure as outlined by the Flom criteria. Six of the patients who failed to obtain functional cure did achieve a "cosmetic cure" (defined as a final strabismus deviation of 10 prism diopters or less) including five patients with ARC. Orthoptics straightened the eyes of 33 of 42 patients with constant strabismus.

In a subsequent paper, Etting[19] reports on another 86 patients. This sample included patients from 6 to 39 years of age and included 43 esotropes and 30 exotropes. Thirty four of the esotropes were constant at all points while the remainder showed some degree of intermittency. The Flom criteria was again used for the functional success. A cosmetic cure category was utilized with a slightly different definition. A cosmetic cure was defined as a patient having a final angle of deviation less than 15 prism diopters. If the patient entered therapy meeting this criterion, then he had to meet an additional requirement that he demonstrated first, second, and third degree fusion at all points in space even though one eye might be slightly turned with ARC at the conclusion of therapy.

Of the 86 patients, 61 achieved functional cure rate while 16 achieved the cosmetic cure. For an overall functional cure rate of 71% and cosmetic cure rate of 19%. The combined cure rate was 90%. This very high success rate is probably related to the fact that a criterion for inclusion in the sample was that the patient complete at least 24 one-half hour orthoptic sessions. The average case duration was approximately 48 treatments. The total cure rate combining functional and cosmetic cures as reported by Etting is considerably higher than the cosmetic results reported with surgery.

Etting also states that "the data points out that the acuity in the amblyopic eye responds to treatment, regardless of the age and onset of therapy or the best initial visual acuity in the amblyopic eye. Since many of these patients had, prior to therapy, the good eye directly occluded for longer periods of time by either their optometrists or their ophthalmologists, with no significant improvement, the use of this preliminary treatment regimen as a prognostic tool is very questionable indeed."

In addition, cures were reported in 19 of 21 patients who had prior surgery, 9 of these patients having had multiple surgery up to four times. Fourteen of this group or 66.7% achieved functional cures up to the Flom criteria.

Ludlam,[5] in a carefully described study, reports the results of orthoptics on 149 non-operated, concomitant strabismus patients treated with orthoptics at the Optometric Center of New York. The cure criteria were very carefully specified and were based upon the previously specified Flom criteria[18] to which Ludlam added an additional requirement that there be satisfactory binocular motility in all directions of gaze to achieve functional cure.

A second set of criteria was adopted for the category of "almost cured." In this category, a patient may lack stereopsis, may exhibit strabismus with diplopia up to 5% of the time, and may need larger amounts of prism to maintain comfortable binocular vision. In all other respects, the patient must meet the criteria for the "functional cure.

Categories of "moderate improvement" and "slight improvement ' were adopted for those patients for whom the main improvement was respectively in more than one or only one of the defects associated with the strabismus. The category of "no improvement" was adopted for those patients for whom there was no significant improvement in the strabismus or its associated defects.

Ludlam outlined the intake procedure and clinical management as well as listing the specific treatment procedures that were utilized. The number and variety of orthoptic procedures utilized in the Ludlam study greatly exceeds the number utilized in most other reported papers, encompassing orthoptics of a broad scope based upon a variety of optometric approaches which are currently in use in the area of strabismus orthoptics. The patients were selected from 284 consecutive strabismus patients seen at the Optometric Center of New York. The following criteria for inclusion of the patient in the study were utilized:
1) The patient showed a manifest deviation
2) The deviation did not respond to corrective lenses
3) There had been no prior surgery
4) There was no evidence of a paralyzed muscle
5) The patient attended at least eight treatment sessions

One hundred forty-nine patients met the criteria and were included in the study. Of the remainder, 51 were still in treatment at the time of the report and therefore could not be included in the experimental group, 19 cases had been previously operated on and still presented residual strabismus, eight had muscle paralysis, nine were accommodative esotropias who responded rather quickly to refractive correction and minimal treatment, and 48 patients did not complete seven training visits (of these 48, almost half dropped out after the initial work-up and undertook no treatment at all).

The overall results of training indicated that 49 or 33% of the sample achieved the functional cure according to the Flom criteria. Another 60 or 40% achieved the almost cured category. In the almost cured category, the patients' eyes were straight all the time under ordinary conditions but tended to deviate when the patient was unusually fatigued, ill with fever, or under strong emotional stress. This occurred not more than 5% of the time and was always accompanied by diplopia. Among the moderately improved patients, there were four who showed straight eyes at all times but who could not be included in the cured and almost cured categories because they showed inadequate motor fusion in all directions or a receded near point of convergence. One was perfectly straight but had asthenopia. Combining these four with the cured and almost cured patients indicated an overall result of orthoptics straightening the eyes of 76% of the patients in the sample. 113 patients of the 149 had binocular vision with straight eyes 95% of the time or more upon conclusion of orthoptics.

Ludlam commented that he felt that the results were less than might be expected because the clinical conditions were not optimum. Treatment was conducted in groups with patients receiving a limited amount of individual care; patients were seen by different clinicians at different times who approached the problem somewhat differently; and the overall management of the cases in the clinic surround was poor. Despite this, the results reported are quite impressive.

Hoffman, Cohen, Feuer, and Klayman[20] report on the effectiveness of orthoptic treatment for strabismus done in a private practice. They report on 55 cases of strabismus that could not be corrected with glasses and who had not had prior surgical treatment. They also required that their patients not show any paresis or paralysis and not have anomalous retinal correspondence. Their results were evaluated according to the Flom criteria as modified by Ludlam.[5] They report an overall success ratio of 87.1% utilizing these high standards for success. Their results with periodic and intermittent strabismics were best but constant strabismics showed a 76.5% success ratio with esotropes slightly less efficiently treated than exotropes. Even among the constant esotropes, there was a 74.5% success ratio.

Two optometric studies evaluated long-term success. Weinstein[21] reports on a follow-up study made on 19 patients previously trained at the University of Houston, College of Optometry. These 19 patients represented a group of former strabismic patients who had been treated successfully and who had been dismissed from treatment a year prior to re-evaluation. 84% of the subjects retained their binocular vision for a year after dismissal.

Ludlam and Kleinman[22] in a follow-up study attempted to assess the long-term results of the patients previously reported upon by Ludlam.[13] They contacted the 113 patients whose eyes had been straightened in the original project three to seven years after dismissal from treatment. They were successful in recalling for examination 81 of the original 113. Of the 32 not returning, 25 had moved from the area and could not be located or traced. Of the seven other patients who were located, two were at college at the time of the evaluations, the parents of two reported that they were satisfied with the results and that they did not wish to remind the child that anything had ever been wrong with the eyes, and three others "couldn't be bothered." To evaluate the patients on this follow-up study, Ludlam and Kleinman adopted three criteria:

1) A cosmetic cure was indicated if parent and/or child reported the patient's eyes were and continued to be straight more than 95% of the time and that if an intermittent deviation occurred, the patient was immediately aware of diplopia and recovered instantly. A second requirement was that the re-evaluation disclose heterophoria for both distance and near fixation.

2) A second criterion was a refractive criterion based upon binocular findings evaluated according to Morgan's Table of Expecteds.[23] If the findings all fell within these normal ranges, the patient was considered to have passed the refractive analysis criterion as well as the cosmetic criterion.

3) The Flom criteria[18] was the third criterion.

The 81 cases analyzed this way produced a cosmetic success of 96%. Only three patients had shown regression in their ability to maintain binocular alignment. 91% of the patients passed the refractive criteria. On the basis of the Flom criteria, 62% of the patients were in the functional cure category and 89% of the patients were in the almost cured category. The overall success ratio on this long-term follow-up study indicated 96% of the patients were cosmetically cured; 92% of the patients passed the refractive criteria; and 89% of the patients showed the ability to pass the very rigid Flom criteria for binocular function. Of 35 patients who were reassessed in the long-term study who had previously been recommended for surgery but who had rejected surgery in favor of orthoptic training, 32 of these were rated as long-term cures.

TABLE 2
RESULTS OF OPTOMETRIC ORTHOPTICS

Study	Number of Cases	Cosmetic % Functional Success	% Functional Cure	Cosmetic Success	% Overall Functional % Cosmetic Cure
Layland[16]	107	72	67%	19	85%
Etting[16]	42	27	64%	6	79%
Etting[19]	86	61	71%	16	90%
Ludlam[5] (almost cured and cured both counted as functional result)	149	109	73%	4	76%
Hoffman, et. al.[20]	55	63	87%	-	87%
TOTALS	439	332	76%	44	86%

Differences in results

Although the ophthalmologic-orthoptist cure rates for strabismus of 56% achieving high level functional cures and 67% achieving cosmetic success are impressive figures, the optometric studies show a high level functional cure rate of 76% and almost 86% cosmetic success. While some of this superiority of approximately 20% in favor of optometric orthoptics may be due to case selection in the individual series, this is probably not the prime reason. As a matter of fact, four of the ophthalmologic-orthoptic reports[6,7,8,15] were limited to intermittent and constant exotropia, with a combined functional cure rate of 59% whereas in the optometric reports[5,16,17,19,20] exotropias showed a combined cure rate of 87%.

It was not always possible to ascertain the full treatment protocol from the articles. There did seem to be a trend for optometric orthoptics to involve more active office treatment visits than orthoptic technician orthoptics. This may have contributed somewhat to the difference in cures.

A more likely explanation of the better cure rates is that most optometric orthoptics incorporated a broader approach to orthoptics utilizing many more treatment modalities, techniques, and strategies.

Ludlam,[5] for instance, lists ten hand-eye coordination activities, eight accommodation-convergence training procedures, seven motility training procedures, nineteen techniques for fusion in space, and eleven instrument fusion techniques along with six occlusion techniques. When mentioned at all, most of the ophthalmologic-orthoptist studies report use of only a handful of techniques or instruments.

Orthoptics in optometric education

This great scope of orthoptics is a direct reflection of the training of the optometrist in this area of practice. Indeed, orthoptics is an integral and vital part of optometric practice, generally mentioned in the legal definition of an optometrist among the various states and occupying a significant portion of the professional school training of the optometrist. The pre-professional undergraduate preparation of the optometrist now requires three years, with the vast majority of students entering the professional program with a bachelor degree. A significant portion of the four-year professional program is devoted to preparation of the optometrist to offer orthoptic therapy.

while the didactic sequence varies somewhat among the different colleges of optometry, the overall curriculum content is fairly similar since all optometry colleges now prepare graduates to sit for a National Board Examination. Typical didactic preparation of the optometrist to practice orthoptics can be illustrated by listing those courses (Table 3) in the curriculum at the State College of Optometry, State University of New York,[24] which pertain to this aspect of practice:

TABLE 3		
Course	Lecture Hours	Lab Hours
Gross Human Anatomy	40	40
Ocular Anatomy and Physiology	60	40
Neuroanatomy	30	20
Visual Perception & Information Processing	60	20
Binocular Vision	30	20
Perceptual & Cognitive Development	30	
Behavior Modification	20	10
Introduction to Optometric Theory	40	10
Geometric Optics (including Brewster and Wheatstone stereoscopes)	120	40
Physiological Optics (including oculomotor system and ocular motility)	130	80
Optometric Theory including 40 hours on strabismus and amblyopia	180	
Vision Training (Orthoptics)	90	90

The clinical program in orthoptics and vision training of the State College of Optometry begins in the third professional year. By this time, the students have had extensive clinical exposure in the general optometry clinic and are quite competent at refraction and pathology detection. They have three hours weekly of specific orthoptic clinic in a very closely supervised surround during their entire third year. The faculty/student ratio in this clinic is 1:3. For the entire last year of the professional program (including the summer between the third and fourth academic years), the students are in orthoptic and vision training clinic for nine hours per week. During this period, the students are scheduled to do supervised, in-depth intake orthoptic evaluations on approximately 100 patients. In addition, they manage the treatment of approximately 50 orthoptic patients involving 300 or more patient visits. This clinical exposure is very tightly supervised, maintaining the same 1:3 faculty/student ratio. In addition to orthoptic evaluations and actual administration of orthoptic procedures, the students are also responsible for case summaries and reports, and there are ongoing weekly seminars with senior faculty of the Vision Training Department.

The basic anatomy and physiology of ocular motility and binocular vision become the background for understanding the perceptual aspects of binocular function. Along with this, there are courses in human and perceptual development and behavior modification and learning theory coupled with extensive preparation in the specific procedures of orthoptics and vision training. This culminates in closely supervised clinical instruction on actual patients. It is no wonder then, that optometric orthoptics proves to be successful and that optometrists generally seek and achieve high-level functional results in their therapy.

Orthoptics is a viable treatment modality for strabismus and should be considered as such in its own right. The data presented in the foregoing studies clearly indicates that orthoptics can be successful in any hands. Optometric orthoptics offers *functional* cure rates which exceed the success rate of cosmetic treatment by surgery, with none of the attendant risks[25,26]. It is only proper that patients with strabismus be offered the opportunity to benefit from this bloodless and highly efficient treatment modality in the interests of restoring normalcy to an otherwise defective visual system.

Conclusions

The papers cited here are the results of extensive literature searches. The cited papers have been selected, not because the results were excellent, but rather solely on the basis that:

a) the authors presented sufficient descriptive information on which to base extraction of statistics and,

b) orthoptic training was the only form of therapy used.

Using these criteria, published articles were summarized and the enclosed statistics were compiled. Success rates for functional cure ranged from 56% in the ophthalmologic-orthoptist studies to 76% in the optometric studies. Cosmetic cure rates ranged respectively from 67% to 86%. The reasons for the higher functional and cosmetic cure rates in the optometric studies have been discussed. However, the important point here is that the functional and cosmetic cure rates are extremely impressive for both groups and especially impressive for the optometric studies. It has also been well established that the optometrists are excellently trained and have the appropriate background to administer this form of therapy. Orthoptics is an extremely effective treatment modality and should be available as a readily accessible treatment for strabismus.

Acknowledgement

The authors wish to thank Drs. I. Suchoff, M. Birnbaum and P. Kruger for their assistance.

Footnote

This research project was underwritten in part by grants from the American Optometric Association and from the College of Optometrists in Vision Development.

References

1. Graham PA. Epidemiology of strabismus. Br J Ophth 1974 Mar;58(3):224-231.
2. Roberts J. Eye examination findings among children. 1972 Vital Health Stat 11(115).
3. Roberts J. Eye examination findings among youths 12-17 years. Vital Health Stat 1975;11(155).
4. Lipton EL. A study of the psychological effects of strabismus. Psychoanal Study Child 1970;25:146-74.
5. Ludlam WM. Orthoptic treatment of strabismus. Am J Opt 1961 Jul;38(7):369-88.
6. Chryssanthou G. Orthoptic management of intermittent exotropia. Am Orthopt J 1974;4:69-72.
7. Sanfilippo S, Clahane A. The effectiveness of orthoptics alone in selected cases of exodeviation: The immediate results and several years later. Am Orthopt J 1970;20:104-17.
8. Altizer LB. The non-surgical treatment of exotropia. Am Orthopt J 1972;22:71-6.
9. Gillan RU. An analysis of one hundred cases of strabismus treated orthoptically. Br J Ophth 1945 Aug;29(8):420-28.
10. Guibor GP. Practical details in the orthoptic treatment of strabismus. Arch Ophth 1934 Dec;12(12)887-901.
11. Guibor GP. The possibilities of orthoptic training - further report. Am J Ophth 1934 Sept;17(9):834-9.
12. Guibor GP. Some possibilities of orthoptic training. Arch Ophth 1934 Mar;11(3):433-55.
13. Guibor GP. Early diagnosis and non-surgical treatment of strabismus. Am J Dis Child 1936;52:907-15.
14. Zaki HA. Role of orthoptic exercises alone (without the aid of surgery) in the treatment of small angles of deviation. Bull Ophth Soc Egypt 1972;65:201-04.
15. Cooper EL, Leyman IA. The management of intermittent exotropia: A comparison of the results of surgical and non-surgical treatment. Am Orthopt J 1977;27:61-7.
16. Layland B. An optometric treatment of strabismus. Aust J Optom 1971 Jun;54(6):205-16.
17. Etting G. Visual training for strabismus - success rate in private practice. Optom Wkly 1973;64(48):1172-5.
18. Borish IM. Clinical Refraction, 3 ed. Chicago: Professional Press, 1970:1323-4.
19. Etting GL. Strabismus study -visual therapy in private practice. (submitted for publication, J Am Optom Assoc)
20. Hoffman L, Cohen AH, Feuer G, Klayman I. Effectiveness of optometric therapy for strabismus in a private practice. Am J Optom 1970 Dec;47(12):990-5.
21. Weinstein E. The effectiveness of strabismus training a year after dismissal. Mo Optom 1972 Mar;52(3):10-11.
22. Ludlam WM, Kleinman BI. The long range results of orthoptic treatment of strabismus. Am J Optom 1965 Nov;42(11):647-84.
23. Borish IM. Clinical Refraction:910.
24. State College of Optometry, State University of New York, 1976-1977 catalog.
25. Bietti GB. Problems of anesthesia in strabismus surgery. Int Ophthmol Clin 1966 Fall;6(3):727-37.
26. Dunlap EA. Complications in strabismus surgery .Int Ophthmol Clin 1966 Fall6(3):609-32.

INTERMITTENT EXOTROPIA

Intermittent exotropia has always been of great interest to me. I'm not sure of the exact prevalence, but early in my career, it was estimated at 1%. This is a very significant number of people. Surgery is probably the most frequent treatment despite rather poor success. Optometric treatment is far more successful and it has always bothered me that this has not become the primary treatment modality. As an introduction to one lecture to a general optometric audience a number of years ago, I presented some calculations indicating that if all intermittent exotropes were given proper optometric training, a huge number of patients could enjoy the benefits of normal binocular function without the cosmetic disfigurement of a wandering eye – while at the same time, the optometric manpower need of such a program could immediately absorb all of the graduating seniors from all optometric schools combined. The shame of this is that so few optometric practices treat this condition. The greater pity is that treatment can be so successful.

In 1985, I co-authored a paper surveying the outcomes of surgery. The results are dismal. Only one third of the operated patients achieved normal binocular function and straight eyes, while one sixth of the patients were actually worse off after surgery. These results were compared with results of optometric treatment in a 1986 paper. Both papers are presented here.

The two papers follow.

Results of Surgical Treatment of Intermittent Divergent Strabismus

Nathan Flax*
Arkady Selinow**
Am J Optom Physiol Opt 1985;62(2):100-4 .

Optometrist, M.S., Member of Faculty, FAAO
**Optometrist, Member of Faculty, FAAO*
State College at Optometry, State University at New York, New York, New York

Abstract

Inasmuch as surgery is often suggested as the primary treatment for intermittent exotropia, we undertook an extensive literature search to ascertain the outcome of this treatment. Surprisingly, only 22 papers were located which gave pre-surgical and post-surgical results for intermittent exotropia using reasonably clear success criteria. Many other papers were located but were excluded because they either failed to state the criteria used, lumped exotropia and esotropia together in their reported successes, or used orthoptics along with surgery. The total number of cases reported in the 22 acceptable papers was analyzed in terms of four levels of success to permit comparison across studies. These four levels were: functional success, motor alignment, cosmetically acceptable, and unsuccessful (no change or worse). The data are tabulated and summarized.

Key Words

intermittent exotropia, strabismus surgery results, binocular function

About one-fifth of all strabismics have intermittent exotropias,[1-3] a condition affecting 1% of the population.[4] Intermittent exotropia is usually classified as basic exotropia, convergence insufficiency, or divergence excess based upon Duane's classification.[5] The last category, divergence excess, is further subdivided into "true" and "simulated," a distinction which may influence the particular surgical approach used.[6] This report does not distinguish among the various categories of intermittent exotropia, but rather analyzes the reported results of surgery for all types of intermittent exotropia taken together.

Methods

To accomplish our purpose of analyzing the results of surgery for intermittent exotropia, an extensive literature search was undertaken using *Medlars II* (1967-1980), *Excerpta Medica Ophthalmologica* (1950-1981), *Ophthalmic Literature* (1953-1981), the bibliographies of standard ophthalmologic textbooks,[7,8] and 10 current ophthalmic journals (see Appendix), thus making our search current to December 1982. We sought all papers with pre-surgical and post-surgical results. Papers without clear or adequate descriptions of the success criteria used could not be analyzed and were therefore excluded. Because our interest was in the effectiveness of surgery, we did not use studies in which orthoptics was included in the treatment along with surgery. Inasmuch as the presence of amblyopia, which is not usual in intermittent strabismus, would tend to reduce functional success and thus bias the results against a good clinical outcome, we omitted all amblyopic subjects from our analysis. For similar reasons we excluded any patient who had had extraocular muscle surgery before becoming part of the studied clinical population, although patients who began as intermittent exotropes and then received multiple surgeries were included. This avoided contamination with patients who had previously had surgery for another condition which then resulted in intermittent exotropia. A total of only 22 papers[3,6,9-28] were located which met the minimum scientific standard of giving pre-surgical and post-surgical results using clearly stated success criteria.

Most of the literature search citations that dealt with the results of surgery could not be analyzed due to one or more of the following reasons: (1) No criteria were used (i.e., the results were reported as "80% were successful" with no statement of what constituted success). (2) Esotropia and exotropia were not separated. (3) Results were stated as averages of all deviations (i.e., average preoperative angle 40 prism diopters and average postoperative angle 10 prism diopters with no statement of the results on individual cases). (4) Exophorias were not differentiated from exotropias.

In several papers, where the purpose was the comparison of orthoptics vs. surgery, only the surgically treated cases were considered. This left a total of 1490 patients described in 22 different studies. Insofar as we can determine, we have included every credible paper in the ophthalmic literature over the past 30 years that has reported on the outcome of purely surgical treatment of intermittent exotropia.

Criteria for Analysis of Data

To permit aggregating data across studies, we have adopted four criteria. These are functional success, motor alignment, cosmetically acceptable, and unsuccessful. The descriptions of these categories are:

1. Functional success requires that the post-surgical patient demonstrates no tropia at any distance by cover test, motor fusion ranges at distance and near as tested by prisms or in an amblyoscope, and sensory fusion. It should be mentioned that the functional success criteria we had to adopt in order to permit any useful analysis was far less stringent than the functional success criteria used in the reporting of orthoptic results.[25]

2. Motor alignment requires that the post-surgical patient demonstrates no acceptable tropia at any distance by cover test, with no demonstration of sensory improvement.

3. Cosmetically acceptable requires that the post-surgical patient demonstrates a strabismus which measures less than 15 prism diopters. No functional binocularity need be present. (A number of patients were converted from intermittent strabismics to low-angle constant strabismics. Although these are considered to be cosmetic successes for the purposes of this study, in these instances the benefits to the patients may be questionable.)

4. Unsuccessful cases did not meet any of the three prior category criteria or were unchanged or worse after surgery. It was not always possible to differentiate between non-improvement and worsening of the condition because of the method of data presentation.

Data Analysis

Five studies[13-15,20,24] reported data in a manner permitting analysis of functional success. (The others did not give functional results after surgery.) This combined group of 571 patients is summarized in Table 1. In this group 34.3% were functionally successful, 27.5% were motorically aligned, and 16.3% were cosmetically acceptable. An aggregate percentage of 78.1% were cosmetically acceptable or better,

TABLE 1. Functional results of surgical treatment of intermittent exotropia.					
Author	Number	Functional	Motorically Aligned*	Cosmetically Aligned*	Unsuccessful*
Cooper and Leyman[13]	264	110	109	-	45
Dunlap and Gaffney[14]	100	12	21	24	43
Folk[15]	50	14	27	-	9
Moore[20]	57	19	-	29	9
Pratt-Johnson et al[24]	100	41	-	40	19
Total	571	196 (34.3%)	157 (27.5%)	93 (16.3%)	125 (21.9%)

see text for specific definitions of criteria

with less than one-half of these patients showing good binocular function post-surgically. The remainder were either left with a post-surgical deviation greater than 15 prism diopters, unimproved, or were worse after surgery.[Table 1]

The remaining 17 studies could be analyzed on the basis of the motor alignment of the eyes, but not function, because they did not provide postoperative fusion measurements. These studies, which involved a total of 919 patients, are summarized in Table 2. Of this group, 42.0% achieved elimination of the strabismus, 15.8% were cosmetically acceptable, and the remaining 42.2% were not cosmetically acceptable.

Combining the results shown in Tables 1 and 2 discloses that 977 of 1490 (65.6%) patients operated on for intermittent divergence excess achieved a cosmetically acceptable end result. Of these, it seems probable that approximately one-half were no longer strabismic on cover test after surgery. The remaining one-third of the entire sample did not achieve even the minimum benefit of being left with a cosmetically acceptable deviation.

Most authors did not present their data in a way which permitted differentiation between patients who were improved cosmetically (although not sufficiently improved to be considered successful) and patients who were unchanged, or worse after surgery than they were before. In a number of studies the presence of cases damaged by surgery is evident. For instance, Moore[20] discussed patients who ended with "grossly over-corrected" esotropia; 43% of Dunlap and Gaffney's[14] patients ended up with one of the following: exotropia of greater than 20 prism diopters at distance, esotropia of greater than 10 prism diopters at distance and near, or esophoria of greater than 14 prism diopters at distance and near; Pratt-Johnson, et al.[24] created amblyopia in 4%, exotropia of 35 prism diopters in 2% and induced hypertropia in 18% of their patients; Burian and Spivey[11] reported an induced vertical deviation which was not present preoperatively in 10% of their total sample of 200 intermittent and constant exotropes; and von Noorden[6] (12%) and Velez[27] (32%) created constant strabismus despite the fact that all of their subjects were only intermittently strabismic before surgery. The surgical failures could be analyzed in eight studies[6,10,15-17,20,26,27] involving 393 patients. These data are presented in Table 3. In this group at least 17.6% were not helped at all or were worse after surgery than before.

TABLE 2.
Nonfunctional results of surgical treatment of intermittent exotropia.

Author	Number of cases	Motorically Aligned*	Cosmetically Acceptable*	Unsuccessful*
Ballen[9]	16	12	-	4
Bedrossian[10]	35	24	-	11
Burian and Spivey[11]	98	54	-	44
Clarke and Noel[12]	78	33	-	45
Fletcher and Silverman[3]	60	45	-	15
Gillies[16]	92	24	-	68
Hamtil and Place[17]	9	7	2	0
Hardesty et al[18]	50	39	4	7
Johnson[19]	51	25	20	6
Mulberger and McDonald[21]	25	8	7	10
Mumma[22]	95	30	23	42
Newman and Mazow[23]	30	-	20	10
Raab and Parks[25]	93	-	51	42
Swan[26]	25	6	9	10
Veler[27]	34	14	9	11
von Noorden[6]	91	48	-	43
Windsor[28]	37	17	-	20
Total	**919**	**386 (42.0%)**	**145 (15.8%)**	**388 (42.2%)**

* see text for specific definitions of criteria

The paper by Burian and Spivey[11] is frequently cited and is one of the few which gave extensive pre-surgical functional data. This paper proved difficult to analyze due to the unusual way in which they present their results. By giving only combined group data, it was not possible to ascertain the changes in any single patient. Their functional criteria was stereopsis of 50 to 100%, which 67% of their postoperative patients achieved. Inasmuch as 31% of this sample of intermittent exotropes showed this level of stereopsis before surgery, it would seem that only 36% of the patients improved. It is also possible that these "functional" cures included cases still exotropic but able to demonstrate stereopsis in an amblyoscope, or intermittent strabismics who could demonstrate stereopsis when aligned,[30] a phenomenon characteristic of intermittent exotropia. The peculiarity of their method of presenting the data is attested to by the fact that they report a higher number of functional successes than cosmetic successes. Similarly, we could not include their cosmetic results because their distance and near cover test results are presented separately with no way for the reader to know whether a particular patient was cosmetically straight at all distances. Phorias and tropias were not separated in their cosmetic results. We were able to include this study in our motorically aligned group by extrapolating how many of their patients ended up with phorias post-surgically.

TABLE 3.
No change and/or worse after surgery for intermittent exotropia*

Author	Number of Cases	Worse and/or No Change	Comments
Bedrossian[10]	35	1	No change
Folk[15]	50	0	-
Gillies[16]	92	31	No change
Hamtil and Place[17]	9	0	-
Moore[20]	57	9	No change or grossly overcorrected esotropia
Swan[26]	25	3	No change
Velez[27]	91	14	No change
von Noorden[6]	**393**	**69 (17.6%)**	

See text for explanation

Summary

We have surveyed the literature reporting the outcome of surgery, including multiple operations, as treatment for intermittent exotropia. To permit comparison among studies we have defined a number of success criteria. Each study was analyzed according to these standards. If there was ambiguity as to the appropriate classification, the case was assigned to the higher classification. Cases amblyopic before surgical treatment, secondary exotropes, or consecutive exotropes were not included. Any bias is in the direction of overstating the proportion of successful outcomes.

A surprising number of papers had to be omitted because they failed to meet certain rather basic requirements of scientific writing. They failed to state the criteria used; they used averaged data in a manner that made it impossible to determine the number of patients in each category; they failed to differentiate between phoria and tropia; or did not distinguish between esodeviation and exodeviation. Credible reports involving 1490 patients were located.

One-third of the reported cases did not achieve even the minimum benefit of being left with a low-angle deviation, with the indication that one in six derived absolutely no benefit at all or were harmed by the surgery. Two-thirds did achieve straight eyes, but only one-third attained normal binocular function along with alignment.

Appendix
The 10 current ophthalmic journals are as follows;
Acta Ophthalmologica
American Journal of Ophthalmology
Archives of Ophthalmology
British Journal of Ophthalmology
Documenta Ophthalmologica
Investigative Ophthalmology and Visual Science
Journal of Pediatric Ophthalmology and Strabismus

Ophthalmic Surgery
Ophthalmology (American Academy of Ophthalmology)
Survey of Ophthalmology

References

1. Schlossman A, Boruchof SA. Correlation between physiologic and clinical aspects of exotropia. Am J Ophthalmol 1955;40:53-64.

2. Pickwell LD. Prevalence and management of divergence excess. Am J Optom Physiol Opt 1979;56:78-81.

3. Fletcher MC, Silverman SJ, Strabismus. Part I. A summary of 1110 consecutive cases. Am J Ophthalmol 1966;61:86-94.

4. Borish IM, Clinical Refraction. 3rd ed. Chicago; Professional Press, 1970:1203.

5. Duane A. A new classification of the motor anomalies of the eyes based upon physiological principles, together with their symptoms, diagnosis and treatment. Ann Ophthalmol Otolaryngol 1896;5:969 and 1897;6:84,247.

6. von Noorden GK. Divergence excess and simulated divergence excess: diagnosis and surgical management. Doc Ophthamol 1969;26(71):9-28.

7. von Noorden GK. Burian von Noorden's Binocular Vision and Ocular Motility. St. Louis: CV Mosby, 1980.

8. Hugonnier R, Hugonnier S, Troutman S. Strabismus, Heterophoria, Ocular Motor Paralysis, St. Louis: CV Mosby, 1969.

9. Ballen PH. Surgical treatment of intermittent exotropia. J Pediatr Ophthal 1970;7:55-9.

10. Bedrossian EH. Surgical results following the recession-resection operation for intermittent exotropia. Am J Ophthalmol 1962;53:351-9.

11. Burian HM, Spivey BE. The surgical management of exodeviations. Am J Ophthalmol 1965;59:603-20.

12. Clarke WN, Noel LP. Surgical results in intermittent exotropia. Can J Ophthalmol 1981;16:66-9.

13. Cooper EL, Leyman IA. The management of intermittent exotropia. A comparison of the results of surgical and non-surgical treatment. In: Moore S, Mein J, Stockbridge L, eds. Orthoptics: Past, Present and Future. New York: Stratton Intercontinental Medical Book Corporation, 1976:563-8.

14. Dunlap EA, Gaffney RB. Surgical management of intermittent exotropia. Am Orthopt J 1963;13:20-33.

15. Folk ER. Surgical results in intermittent exotropia. Arch Ophthalmol 1956;55:484-7.

16. Gillies WE. The results of treatment of intermittent exodeviation. Trans Aust Coll Ophthalmol 1970;2:100-5.

17. Hamtil LW. Place KC. Review of surgical results using bilateral lateral rectus recession for the correction of exodeviations. Ann Ophthalmol 1978;10:1731-4.

18. Hardesty HH, Boynton JR, Keenan JP. Treatment of intermittent exotropia. Arch Ophthalmol 1978;96:268-74.

19. Johnson DS. Some observations on divergence excess. Arch Ophthalmol 1958;60:7-11.

20. Moore S. Orthoptic treatment for intermittent exotropia. Am Orthopt J 1963;13:14-20.

21. Mulberger RD, McDonald PR. Surgical management of nonparalytic exotropia. Arch Ophthalmol 1954;52:664-8.

22. Mumma JV. Surgical treatment of exotropia. Am Orthopt J 1975;25:96-100.

23. Newman J, Mazow ML. Intermittent exotropia. Is surgery necessary? Ophthal Surg 1981;12:199-202.

24. Pratt-Johnson JA, Banow JM, Tiulson G. Early surgery for intermittent exotropia. Am J Ophthalmol 1977;84:689-94.

25. Raab EL, Parks MM. Recession of the lateral recti. Arch Ophthalmol 1975;93:584-6.

26. Swan KC. Surgery for exotropia: fusional ability and choice of procedure. Am J Ophthalmol 1960:50:1158-67.

27. Velez G. Results in exotropia. In: Moore S, Mein J, Stockbridge L, eds. Orthoptics: Past, Present and Future. New York: Stratton Intercontinental Medical Book Corporation, 1976:559-62.

28. Windsor CE. Surgery, fusion, and accommodative convergence in exotropia. J Pediatr Ophthalmol 1971;8:166-70.

29. *Flax N, Duckman RH. Orthoptic treatment of strabismus. J Am Optom Assoc 1978:49:1353-61.*
30. *Costenbader FD. The physiology and management of divergent strabismus. In: Allen JH, ed. Strabismus Ophthalmic Symposium 1, St. Louis: CV Mosby, 1950:349-76.*

A Comparison of Functional Results in Intermittent Divergent Strabismus Treated Surgically and Optometrically*

Nathan Flax, O.D.**
J Opt Vis Dev 1986;17:18-9

Dr. Flax has been among the foremost practitioners in vision therapy for over thirty years. During that period of time lie has maintained a specialized practice limited to vision therapy in association with Dr. AM. Rappaport. He has written extensively on the subjects of strabismus and on the relationship between vision and learning. For the past fifteen years he has divided his time between private practice and the State College of Optometry of the State University of New York where he directs the Vision Training Education and Services, holding the rank of professor. Throughout his career he has lectured widely and has been active in optometric organizations. He was a co-founder of the Diplomate Program in Binocular Vision and Perception of the American Academy of Optometry and has received the Skeffington Award from COVD.

*Presented at the Skeffington Symposium, Washington, D.C., January 26-28, 1985.
**FCOVD, FAAO, Professor, State College of Optometry, State University of New York.

Abstract
The literature was reviewed to determine functional outcomes when intermittent exotropia is treated surgically. Twenty-two credible papers were located and these were analyzed in terms of binocular function. The results achieved surgically are compared and contrasted with published results when strabismus is treated orthoptically. The data indicate that vision therapy is most successful than surgery for: intermittent exotropia from both a functional arid cosmetic standpoint.

Introduction

Intermittent exotropia is a condition which affects approximately one percent of the population. Flax and Selenow[1] have conducted an extensive literature search to document functional outcomes of surgery utilized to treat this condition. An attempt was made to locate all papers giving pre-surgical and post-surgical results which could he analyzed in terms of the patient's functional binocularity. Surprisingly, a total of only twenty-two papers could be located in the ophthalmic literature which met the minimum scientific criteria of giving pre and post-surgical results utilizing clearly stated success criteria. Most papers had to be rejected simply because the author gave no indication at all of the success criteria used. Often, esotropia and exotropia, or phorias and tropias, were all lumped together. In a number of instances the results were given as average deviations of an entire sample not permitting any insight at all into what happened to individual cases. The twenty-two papers, which permitted analysis, represent the total number of credible reports in the past thirty years of ophthalmological literature.

Results

Even among the papers selected for analysis, the results were often rather poorly specified. It was impossible to apply any rigorous criteria for functional success similar to the Flom criteria (most often utilized in optometric research). To permit analysis of data, Flax and Selenow adopted four criteria as follows:

1. *Functional success:* the post-surgical patient demonstrated no tropia by cover test, motor fusion ranges at distance and near, and sensory fusion of any kind. This success criteria was far less stringent than those usually used to report orthoptic results.

2. *Motor alignment:* the post-surgical patient demonstrated no tropia by cover test, without sensory improvement.

3. *Cosmetically acceptable:* the post-surgical patient was left with a strabismus which measured less than fifteen prism diopters. No functional binocularity had to be demonstrated.

4. *Unsuccessful:* cases did not it meet any of the three prior criteria and were unchanged or worse after surgery.

In each instance, Flax and Selenow placed the patient in the higher category when the case was borderline between two categories. It might be noted that a number of patients who were placed into the cosmetically acceptable category actually were converted from intermittent strabismus prior to surgery to constant low angle strabismus after surgery. This is a dubious improvement at best.

Five studies involving 571 patients permitted analysis of functional success. The other studies generally did not report functional results after surgery. A total of 34.3% of the patients were functionally successful, 27.5% were motor aligned, and 16.3% were cosmetically acceptable. Summing up, 78.1% of the patients analyzed were cosmetically acceptable or better but only one-half of these showed good binocular function after surgery. The remainder of the cases (21.9%) were left either with a post-surgical deviation greater than fifteen prism diopters, showed no improvement at all, or were actually worse after surgery.

The remaining seventeen studies involving 919 patients could be analyzed on the basis of motor alignment but not function since insufficient data on fusion was presented. Of these, 42.0% of the patients achieved elimination of the strabismus, 15.8% were cosmetically acceptable, and the remaining 42.2% were unsuccessful.

Combining all of the groups indicates that 977 (65.6%) of 1,490 patients operated on for intermittent divergent excess achieved a cosmetically acceptable end result. Of these, approximately one half were no longer strabismic on cover test after surgery. One third of the entire sample did not achieve even the minimum benefit of being left with cosmetically acceptable eyes.

A number of papers disclosed that many patients were actually unimproved or worse after surgery. Among the results encountered were instances of "grossly over-corrected" esotropia, exotropia greater than 20 prism diopters at distance, esotropia of greater than 10 prism diopters at distance and near, esophoria of greater than 14 prism diopters at distance and near, amblyopia, exotropia of greater than 35 prism diopters, and induced hypertropia. In several instances, constant exotropes were created out of intermittents. It was possible to analyze the surgical failures in eight studies involving 393 patients. This data indicates at least 17.6% of the patients were clearly not helped at all or worse after surgery.

Summary

This literature review by Flax and Selenow indicates that functional results were obtained in only one third of the patients operated on for intermittent exotropia. The success criteria used for the ophthalmological studies was significantly lower than those characteristically used for studies reported in the orthoptic literature or the optometric literature. Despite using lower standards, the reported results are significantly poorer.

In a previous paper by Flax and Duckman[2], the results of orthoptic intervention in strabismus were also discussed in functional terms. In this paper, rather high and quite acceptable success criteria were utilized both optometrically and orthoptically. While the Flax-Duckman paper did not specifically analyze intermittent exotropia, the overall success rates were 56% functional cure and 67% cosmetic cure when treatment was solely orthoptics done by orthoptic technicians. When the treatment was offered by optometrists, the functional cure rate was 76'% and the cosmetic rate was 86%. It should be noted that the orthoptic and optometric results reported by Flax and Duckman included all types of strabismus, many of which had a poorer prognosis than intermittent exotropia. Within these studies, the success rate for intermittent exotropes generally approached or exceeded the 90% level.

One study that was included in both the Flax and Selenow paper and the Flax and Duckman paper was that of Cooper and Leyman.[3] This study compared surgical and non-surgical treatments with the non-surgical treatment done by orthoptic technicians. The functional cure rate was 59% with orthoptics and 42% with surgery.

In summary, these literature searches indicate that optometrists produce high level binocular cures among intermittent exotropes a much greater percentage of the time than surgeons can produce only cosmetic improvement. At least 86% (and probably more than 90%) of intermittent exotropes treated optometrically become straight-eyed and can demonstrate binocular function using rigorous criteria. In contrast only 34% of operated cases demonstrate less rigorous binocular function, and only 65.6% of operated patients demonstrate a cosmetically acceptable end result. Additionally, one in six operated patients demonstrates no change or is actually worse after the surgery. Clearly then, vision therapy should be the initial mode of treatment for intermittent exotropia, with surgery reserved for those patients unresponsive to vision therapy.

References

1. *Flax N, Selenow A. Results of surgical treatment of intermittent divergent strabismus. Am J Optom 1962;2:100-4.*
2. *Flax N, Duckman R.,Orthoptic treatment of strabismus. J Am Optom Assoc.1978;49:1353-61.*
3. *Cooper EL, Leyman LD. The management of intermittent exotropia: A comparison of the results of surgical and non surgical treatment. In: Moore S, Main J, Stockbridge L, eds. Orthoptics: Past, Present and Future. New York: Stratton Intercontinental Medical Book Corp., 1976:563-8.*

A TREATMENT APPROACH FOR INTERMITTENT EXOTROPIA

A 90% success rate for optometric training was the figure used in the data extrapolated in a 1986 paper comparing vision therapy to surgery for treatment of intermittent exotropia. Actually, I feel that the success rate in this type of strabismus should be almost 100% when dealing with cases which meet the criteria for divergence excess. In over forty years of practice, anything less than full resolution of this type of strabismus was rare. Very early in my career, influenced by the thinking of Fred Brock (a true pioneer who seems to be disappearing from optometric memory) I developed a different approach to training this condition. I began lecturing about this approach in the early 1960s. The earliest record I can find is a 1963 presentation at what was then called the Eastern Seaboard Vision Training Conference (now called KISS – Kraskin Invitational Skeffington Symposium) Another early document is the transcript of the 25th San Jose Vision Training Seminar in 1968. Both of these are transcripts of oral presentations. They give insight into the evolution of the approach as well as specific training procedures, and are included here with minimal editing . These early presentations discuss the comparison of the divergence excess patient to the OEP-Skeffington B case type and the utilization of near plus for long term stability. In 1996, I published a more formal paper. While more succinct, the last paper does not detail specific training procedures.

The transcripts and paper follow.

The Optometric Training of Intermittent Divergent Strabismus

Nathan Flax, O.D.
Presented at Eastern Seaboard Vision Training Conference, 1963
Washington, DC

This paper will concern itself with that form of intermittent divergent strabismus known as divergence excess. In this type of strabismus the angle of deviation is greater at distance than it is at near. Generally, the patient exhibits an intermittent exotropia at far and straight eyes at near point. The prognosis in this condition has not been particularly good. Surgery is generally ineffective since the concept of muscle weakness falls down completely when one considers that these patients are usually capable of a normal near point of convergence. The results with standard orthoptic training have likewise not been terribly effective. It is possible to build enormous induction ranges and yet the patient still manifests a periodic exotropia at far point.

This type of strabismus has also been labeled inattention strabismus. Many intermittent exotropes function binocularly whenever the task demand requires the two eyes be used and they are concentrating on the activity at hand. They tend to go into the strabismic position when they are not paying attention to anything such as when they are day dreaming. They may frequently close one eye, particularly in bright light.

A patient with divergence excess strabismus seems to intuitively analyze an activity and selects the mode of response in accordance with the requirements of the task. They seem to have a dual pattern of performance. When necessary, they can and do function binocularly with a high level of integration and are able to demonstrate good quality stereopsis. On the other hand, when there is no particular need to operate binocularly they will often revert to a rather deep suppression. When gazing into the far distance, binocular vision and stereopsis are of relatively little importance and they will let an eye wander. When engaged in a near task requiring stereopsis, they will bifixate and show good stereopsis. Some will show a receded near point of convergence when asked to look at a muscle light and not become aware of diplopia. When they are asked to touch the light, the eyes converge properly. The additional element imposed by the requirement to touch the object of regard seems to trigger the correct binocular response.

In usual strabismus training, the patient is expected to go through the stages of simultaneous binocular awareness, flat fusion, and stereopsis. These are referred to as first, second, and third degree fusion, implying a hierarchical relationship. Indeed many strabismus training programs follow just such a sequence. The question arises as to the appropriateness of this model for the divergence excess patient who shows best binocular integration and alignment when the task requires stereopsis. They will posture their eyes in a straight position when the information from the task necessary to achieve at the task can only be obtained when two eyes are being used simultaneously and let an eye drift when the task presented can be accomplished monocularly. The order of difficulty for a patient with divergence excess strabismus might be stereopsis, flat fusion, and lastly simultaneous binocular perception – a reversal of the traditional first, second and third degree fusion concept.

The ultimate goal in training must be development of easily maintained binocular alignment under conditions demanding minimal attention or stereopsis. It is not sufficient that the patient be able to use two eyes together when necessary. The patient must be able to maintain straight eyed posture and binocular alignment even in the face of a low level task demand so that this patient will not revert to the periodic strabismus when daydreaming. This need to develop binocular posturing, independent of a need for simultaneous use of information from the two eyes, causes me to re-assess the possible mechanisms for maintaining straight eyes. Traditionally, it is assumed that a person maintains straight eyes in order to avoid diplopia. If this was the primary means by which we maintain straight eyes, we might expect to hear patient reports of diplopia followed by fusion, particularly for those with high phorias. This is not often reported. The intermittent exotrope aligns his eyes not to avoid diplopia but rather to utilize the benefits of fusion and stereopsis. This individual can demonstrate a high level of binocular function and still shift in and out of a relatively deep suppression. While making the patient aware of diplopia when the eye diverges can be utilized with reasonable success, my treatment approach is based upon directly developing the ability to maintain alignment even under conditions which do not require binocular function. I believe that this approach gives more lasting cures.

A possible mechanism to cue alignment is proprioceptive awareness of eye position. Cultivation of this mechanism brings strongly to the forefront the need for monocular procedures in the treatment of such a problem. Monocular procedures emphasizing proprioception are exceedingly useful in a training program to overcome divergence excess. Particularly helpful is the use of prism saccadic training. When a loose prism is suddenly introduced on a monocular basis while the patient is fixating a distant target, many strabismics make the necessary eye movement to pick up fixation, but do not seem to register the movement. they are unaware of any appearance of the target moving. Sometimes, they will not appreciate apparent target movement of even a 5 or 10 prism diopter shift of eye position. It is as if there is a dead zone. With training, most patients eventually appreciate as little as ½ prism diopter shifts.

Treatment begins with pursuit and saccadic training on a monocular basis, while also utilizing peripheral binocular activities. The recommended procedure is to operate at two levels of training simultaneously. Monocular training procedures are done to create proprioceptive awareness, while at the same time peripheral binocular training is done to insure the patient's ability to continue to function in a binocular fashion. The binocular training at this phase of treatment should studiously avoid any attempt at foveal or central work. The binocular training should begin peripherally and should involve the utilization of stereoscopic targets from the outset. All training should be done with the patient posturing in a straight position rather then at the angle of squint.

This is important since we must recognize that such a patient has the ability to operate binocularly in those very task situations which require three dimensional judgments which can only be made on the basis of two eyes operating simultaneously. It therefore becomes necessary to begin at the point where the patient can operate most efficiently and to cultivate this before attempting to move the patient into other areas of function. It is also important to avoid training at the angle of squint since the ultimate goal of training will be to have the patient learn to match the proprioceptive awareness of where his eyes are when they are functioning correctly with the reinforcement that comes from the successful completion of a binocular task. Working at the angle of squint will tend to negate this approach since there will be a report of binocular function in a situation where the proprioceptive signals from the extra ocular muscles will not represent straight eyed posturing.

Such a training program for peripheral binocular function is generally best started at either near point or at an intermediate distance utilizing projected anaglyphs or projected vectographs. Projected anaglyphs might be the target material of preference since it is possible to present very simple material in an easily controlled situation. Another advantage to the use of projection material is that it gives the patient an opportunity to stand and move during the course of the binocular training so that the reinforcement of total body kinesthesia ii available. It also is possible to have the patient match the kinesthetic and tactual aspects of the training program with verbal description of what is being seen. The utilization of projection targets also permits the patient to become aware of his surrounds and to work in real space while at the same time avoiding central critical stimulation. This avoidance of central critical stimulation perhaps should be amplified.

In tracing the early development of binocular function, it becomes apparent that the infant begins to learn binocular posturing before that period in development where he might be capable of critical central acuity. In other words, binocular posturing apparently precedes clear seeing. In an attempt to develop proper binocular function, it would seem desirable to follow, insofar as possible, the normal sequence of development. Still another reason why one would want to avoid critical central stimulation is the fact that the intermittent exotrope tends to operate quite satisfactorily on the basis of critical demand but has greater difficulty in operating at the level of minimal demand. It becomes the task of the training situation to foster binocular posturing in the face of a non-critical central demand.

It is not necessary during this phase of training to think of development of fusional ranges. Typically, the patient with divergence excess strabismus can exhibit a reasonable fusion range when the target demand is appropriate. His greatest problem is maintaining binocular posturing in the absence of demand. It is more important that he be taught to integrate general body and ocular kinesthesia with maintenance of straight eyes than it is to insure that he can function binocularly to do a specific highly discrete task.

At the same time the peripheral binocular training is done, some amount of central stimulation may be necessary in certain cases. In those instances where it is not possible to maintain binocular posturing for long enough periods of time to do effective training as has been described in the previous paragraphs, it may be necessary to resort to central stimulation in order to develop more stable posturing. When this is done, such training should be done in a real situation rather than an instrument situation so that there can be the immediate reinforcement by movement and kinesthesia. An excellent training activity for this purpose is the utilization of stick-in-straw procedures. This type of training insures that the patient functions binocularly in a real life situation and can obtain kinesthetic reinforcement for the value judgments made on the basis of visual data. In this particular procedure the patient is permitted to operate at a tactual-visual level. The ultimate goal is to transform this functioning into a visual-tactual performance. This transformation can be expedited by incorporating verbal commands to the trainer so that the examiner's hands can begin to substitute for the patient's hands. In other words, the patient can be asked to use his visual input to direct verbal commands to operate someone else's hands. Such training is quite effective in bridging the gap between the tactual and visual phases of performance.

The work with projected anaglyphs or projected vectographs should also incorporate this verbal phase by having the patient describe SILO and parallax as he moves about. Here, too, there is a marvelous opportunity to have the patient incorporate verbal concepts to match with visual inputs. It is also possible in this training situation to ask the patient to make spatial localization judgments which require him to operate other motor systems on the basis of visual information without the possibility of tactual reinforcement. When the patient reaches that stage in treatment where he can hold a finger or a pointer up to a place in space and say that is where the object seems to be even though he cannot get the tactual reinforcement by feeling the object, the patient has demonstrated his ability to operate on a visual basis. Naturally, the projected anaglyph or vectograph training proceeds through levels of complexity by gradually introducing more complicated targets and by gradually moving from peripheral targets into more central targets. Initially, the patient may he made aware of only one aspect of the situation such as the spatial movement of the target. Ultimately he is asked to become aware of the spatial movement and to incorporate this into SILO. After this, the concept of parallax might be introduced followed by the concept of spatial localization and then ultimately followed by the concept of verbal description. Along with these modifications in task demand, the actual geometry of the task be modified *by* operating at varying distances.

Only after the patient is able to demonstrate parallel eye posture should "regular orthoptics" be undertaken. Antisuppression training should wait until such time that the patient is able to keep his eyes parallel most of the time. Introduction of antisupression training too early in the training program is apt to make the patient aware of diplopia in space when his eye does deviate. This is not apt to serve as a mechanism to hold him straight but is rather apt to serve as an irritant and perhaps may even interfere with establishment of binocular posturing. Similarly, development of better fusional quality and ranges of fusion should wait until the patient is able to demonstrate parallel posturing most of the time. There is no point in putting such a patient into instrument to develop quality of fusion or to do antisuppression training in a deviating position. This would not permit the match between proper binocular function and proper proprioceptive awareness of eye position that is the goal of the training. When instrument training is begun, it should be possible to begin such training at orthophoria or very close to orthophoria rather than in a divergent position. Here again, the training should proceed from the use of stereoscopic target material back through flat fusion material and ultimately into simultaneous binocular perception material. The final stages of such training should be concerned with developing of ranges of posturing on simultaneous perception material. The example of this might be to have the patient keep a star in a circle in a Rotoscope even when base out prism is introduced. Another technique at this point might he the utilization of the Brock posture box where there is a low order fusion demand and where the primary requirement of the task is to maintain parallel posturing of the eyes.

The divergence excess strabismic has his greatest problem in maintaining parallel posture in the face of low order visual demands. He tends to function best at high order three dimensional task than he does at those situations which do not require simultaneous use of both eyes. Therefore the training situation should flow in that direction and ultimately require that the patient posture in the face of a minimal stimulation to binocular function.

Along with the training procedures already outlined, there is yet another approach that is exceedingly valuable in the handling of intermittent exotropia. Plus lenses have an important role in the handling of this optometric problem. Accommodative facility training should be introduced early in the program with particular emphasis upon developing the plus end of the range. This is best understood when we analyze the divergence excess syndrome and realize that, regardless of etiology, the syndrome closely resembles a deeply imbedded OEP "B" problem. Although one might question the instigating factor since most cases of divergence excess appear very early in life prior to the time that cultural near point demands should have had their impact, the similarity in the divergence excess and B case type is striking. As a matter of fact, it is not unusual and almost expected that every divergence excess strabismic goes through a stage where a measurable esophoria is demonstrated at near point. Certainly, by definition, the fact that there is always a greater exophoria at far than there is at near makes one immediately suspicious of a B syndrome.

The use of plus lenses in the case of divergence excess has to be handled quite carefully. Application of plus too soon may have an adverse effect since some of these patients must make use of accommodative convergence at the outset in order to keep their eye postured binocularly. Inhibition of this accommodative convergence too early may make maintenance of binocular function in a parallel position too difficult and may stand in the way of a successful result. However, once the patient can demonstrate binocular function in parallel position with reasonable stability, it becomes valuable to gradually introduce plus lenses with the dual purpose of initially inhibiting accommodation and then ultimately increasing the plus sufficiently so that the patient is asked to function binocularly despite poor acuity. In the latter stages of training, the procedure should be done through high plus which precludes anything but very poor acuity at the training task.

Once the near point esophoria emerges and near point plus acceptance has been developed to a high enough degree, then prescription of plus for near activities in bifocal form becomes a very useful adjunct to the training program. When used in this manner, it is necessary that this plus be given in bifocal form. The case must be treated primarily an a B2 problem. This is almost always the case. Almost without exception divergence excess strabismus cases go through a stage where the induction finding at near is considerably higher than the outduction finding and where an esophoria pattern emerges at near. This is the opportune time to treat them as a B2 and to prescribe in that fashion.

The use of this lens approach has the long term effect of ultimately stabilizing the problem. This is demonstrated by frequent gradual reduction in the far point exophoria over a span of years long after the actual training program has been completed. Along with the reduction of far point exophoria comes a reduction in the far point base in duction finding. This seems to parallel the reduction in the far point exophoria and would seem to indicate that the application of near point plus has served to relieve a stressor agent. Regardless of the actual etiology of divergence excess strabismus the clinical management of the case dictates that it be treated as if it were an embedded B2 case.

It is worth noting that throughout the entire training program there is little if any need to actually train convergence as such. The key to the successful management of the divergence excess patient is to initially train out of instrument in those tasks where the "task analysis" done by the patient requires that be respond to the task binocularly. It is also important that such training be done in a situation where eyes can be maintained in a proper parallel posture so that there can be a matching of the visual data with proper kinesthetic proprioceptive awareness of extra ocular position.

The training program should begin with stereopsis and then ultimately move in the direction of simultaneous perception. It should begin out of instrument and then ultimately move into instrument so that there is a reduction of environmental cues with no possibility of tactual or kinesthetic reinforcement and yet with a need to posture the eyes in a proper position with very few confirming feedback signals from other sensory motor systems. It is also important that plus lenses be used judiciously, initially as a training device and then ultimately prescribed for all near point activity in bifocal form. With such a training and lens approach, intermittent exotropia can be successfully managed.

Training Intermittent Exotropes

Nathan Flax, O.D.
25th Annual San Jose Vision Training Seminar
August 23 - 25, 1968
This was edited from a transcription of the meeting.

For the moment I will limit myself to a discussion of intermittent exotropia of the divergence excess type. The majority of exotropes you will encounter are in this category. These are for the most part periodic intermittent exotropes with better binocular function at near than at far and higher exophoria at far than at near. They are sometimes labeled "inattention strabismus". The youngster daydreams and the eyes wander. They very often, but not always, show an early onset, with the condition presenting anywhere from a year to eighteen months of life. Sometimes, the deviation firs appears after the start of school at ages 7 to 10. The key characteristic an intermittent turn with better binocular function at near than at far.

Utilizing standard orthoptics does not produce very good results (although far better than surgical results).. If you read the orthoptic literature you will find they indicate they are relatively powerless in training intermittent exotropia. They are capable of building fantastic induction ability, but don't do much about the individual's exotropia. Surgery in these cases is notoriously ineffective. although it is repeatedly done. The youngster will frequently go right back to the same divergence after surgery. Our results in this type of case have been uniformly excellent, and I think we are doing things a little bit differently which accounts for this.

I would like to give you an approach to the handling of this type of strabismus that has an ingredient which is a bit different, but quite consistent with a functional analysis of the patient's utilization of the information he gets from his eyes. Some of the things we do in training, which are correctly sequenced for a particular theoretical model, are not necessarily sequenced for the way intermittent exotropes operate. Standard orthoptic approaches categorize three stages of binocular fusion called first degree fusion or simultaneous binocular awareness, second degree or flat fusion, and third degree or stereopsis. The labeling implies a hierarchical sequence which is inappropriate for the divergence excess strabismic.

As I said yesterday, I think in terms of the task analysis. What type of visual function might relate to a particular activity. I think the intermittent exotrope is a master of this concept of task analysis, although it is not done consciously. If you watch the behavior of the intermittent exotrope you will note that generally when there is an advantage to binocular vision, they use it, and when there is no particular advantage they may or may not use it. Characteristically. if you give them spatial manipulation test requiring near point stereopsis, such as placing a stick into a straw, they converge and function binocularly. If the strabismus condition has degenerated sufficiently there may a deterioration of binocular function at near point also, with difficulty in convergence.. In the early stages of the problem convergence is excellent. A little bit later, it. begins to drop off. Even at that point where convergence becomes weak, if you watch these patients carefully on a stick and straw test, you will may see a pulling in of the eyes briefly with a momentary posturing of the eyes at the task, apparently enough to get cues to where the thing straw is located Then they will deviate again while making an excellent stereoscopic placement of the stick into the straw.

If you want to precipitate the maximum turn, have them fixate something beyond 20 feet if you can possibly set it up, say at 30 or 40 feet and ask them to fixate something at the limit of their resolution. Under these circumstances you will precipitate the highest angle of turn. This happens to be a task where binocular vision is of little or no benefit to them. They seem to function in the way best for both worlds. When it is better and more convenient to be binocular, they function binocularly. When there is little advantage to being binocular, they don't bother. In general they are people who are relatively symptom free, most of them are quite happy children, it is the parent who is disturbed when they see the eye wandering. Occasionally it does interfere athletically and scholastically, but usually the degree of interference in their performance is not commensurate with the cosmetic aspects of the problem. They seem to know whether or not the task you give them requires the use of two eyes. The chief complaint that brings them to examination is concern about appearance rather than asthenopia.

This dictates one of the first differences in my training program. I start backwards. Binocular training begins with stereoscopic cards and targets; not with flat fusion targets; not with simultaneous perception targets. The training begins with target materials that require fusion and stereopsis, rather than following the traditional sequence of simultaneous perception, fusion without stereopsis and then stereopsis - a reversal of the standard order.

A second difference is that, insofar as is possible, all binocular training is done with the eyes in alignment. I do not want to develop fusion with the eyes in a deviated position and then gradually develop fusional vergence. Bear in mind that these intermittent exotropes have the ability to align and fuse *before* you begin treatment. Their problem is loss of alignment under conditions which do not favor binocularity.

A rule of thumb which we follow in the handling of the divergent excess strabismic is that we do not do any closed instrument techniques until the individual can posture his eyes straight ahead. We do no training at the objective angle. As I view it, the problem of the exotrope is not a problem of an inability to use both eyes together, but an inability to posture both eyes in a straight ahead position in the absence of a high demand for using both eyes. His is a posturing problem as contrasted to a binocular function problem. He can function binocularly, and often does. His problem is that he cannot persist in maintaining the two eyes in a straight ahead, aligned position when the task does not require it of him. This is the reason most of his turning is done when he daydreams or views things at far distances. Therefore, I am not interested in presenting high level binocular demands to him in his turned position.

Many people have become involved in a controversy of closed instrument versus training in real space. In my opinion both approaches are necessary. Every once in a while optometrists decide to throw out their stereoscopes, etc, because everything has to be done out of instruments. This is utter nonsense. You need both instruments approaches, and non-instrument approaches - particularly for strabismus training. The important thing is to know when you need each modality.

When treating divergence excess intermittent exotropes, I don't do diplopia awareness training. In my opinion it is not an avoidance of diplopia that keeps human eyes straight. If diplopia avoidance was the primary mechanism for maintaining alignment, we should expect brief momentary diplopia to be present in many cases of high phorias. This is not generally the case. While cultivating awareness of diplopia can be used to control the alignment of intermittent exotropes, I believe that this is essentially an artificial mechanism, and a less efficient approach to the treating of the intermittent exotrope. It has been my experience that intermittent exotropes who are trained by methods which emphasize an awareness of diplopia wind up as individuals who can hold their eyes straight when they think about it, but who tend to revert when not concentrating on holding alignment. My job is to teach the patient how to stay straight when not thinking about his eyes; when his eyes are secondary to what he is thinking or doing at the moment, That is when he turns - when he is not paying attention; when he is listening, not looking, when he is thinking, when he is not concentrating on seeing. Therefore anything that insists that he always think about his eyes is doomed to failure. My preference is to train eye proper posture per se.

We do a great deal of training where we intentionally degrade the clarity of the target. The Keystone Overhead Projector with projected anaglyphs becomes the work horse instrument with these people. I daresay every one of these people spend some time each training session using that device. We even did Keystone one better, we threw the machine out of focus intentionally. Very often we will do training with this kind of youngster behind so much plus he can't see clearly, or sometimes throwing the projector out of focus.

A lot of accommodative facility work will be done with all strabismics. In addition to a heavy dose of monocular fixation training, the intermittent exotropes get a heavy dose of accommodative facility training. I can give you some rationale as to why the fixation training and the accommodative training has this impact. In both of these procedures we are making the individual more aware of size and distance relationships while doing these things. If you get right eye to respond to an external stimulus and get left eye to respond to that same stimulus in the same consistent fashion you seem to have a better chance of having right eye respond co jointly with left eye. For whatever reason, a great deal of monocular pursuit, saccadic training and a good deal of accommodative facility training in all of our strabismics.

A question was asked a few minutes ago as to the distance we use with projected anaglyphs. We will begin at that distance where the patient gives me the best and most consistent response. Most of these intermittent exotropes will give you a response to the projected anaglyphs on the first examination, but occasionally you will get one who does not. Then my task is to find some way of developing sufficient binocular alignment to permit me to extend from that arca. I will use devices and combinations of devices. I will use concave lenses if accommodative stimulation will give me sufficient convergence for this person to posture his eyes at a point where I can begin to develop their peripheral fusion. I will make use of stick and straw technique combined with a Brock string to get them to finally posture the eyes. using the stick arid straw as the lever to get them to bring their eyes in, using the Brock string as a means to monitor when they have done this so they can begin to hold the eyes in line. On occasion I will use all three together: minus lenses, stick and straw, and Brock strings.

The patient wears minus lenses. I will use a bare ophthalmoscopic bulb as the muscle light and a drinking straw in the patient's hand. A string is tied to the ophthalmoscope, ready for me to swing in as soon as he gives me binocular posture. I tell him to place the straw, if he makes the correct placement with the eyes coming in at that moment, I push the string in front of him to see if get the awareness of two strings. I am watching his eyes all the time. I may hold it out at the side and put it in, or I may sometimes leave the string there, not questioning about one string or two strings until the eyes come into line. The game is only played when the eyes are in line. As soon as they diverge, no more questions. I don't call the patient's attention to the loss of convergence. When the string V can be maintained, the next step would be to move him in front of near point vectgraphs using the string V while fixating the muscle light to monitor his own eye position while also attending to the vectogram target. When the patient can maintain convergence, the string is removed since this is no longer needed. The training of the divergence excess patient almost always has to begin at near distances because fusion responses are more easily achieved at near.

Training will begin primarily using peripheral stereoscopic targets. The first thing 1 want to be sure of is that they are in fact binocular so I will use what I call a massaging technique. The stereo targets (the best for this purpose are large anaglyph Brock rings) are slowly shifted back and forth between low base in and low base out settings until the patient gives me good indication that he is responding binocularly. I will accept any responses indicative of binocularity, so long as they are consistent. If the patient reports a size change of the ring, or notes movement of the ring closer and further portion. At this juncture, I am not concerned about proper SILO or accurate spatial localization. I just want to be sure that the patient is binocular. I want to be sure that there isn't a lateral shift of the target indicating suppression, or random responses suggesting guessing. When I am sure in my own mind that the patient is binocular, I begin to probe a little bit farther into the quality of the response.

The use of projected anaglyph and vectographic techniques have been largely neglected by optometrists because they felt that there was no good quantifiable ways of controlling them. There are no numbers on a scale when using a device like the Stereomotivator and the doctor is not sure what their patient is supposed to be reporting. Actually, there is no reason why the this is so apparently mysterious. The projected targets should have an appearance of localization in space that is predictable on the basis of very simple geometry. The position at which that target should be seen is a function of the distance from the screen, the patient's interpupillary separation and the disparation of the targets. (Chalkboard work here.) The same holds if we set the instrument for uncrossed or base in disparity, they project beyond the plane of projection and where the lines of sight cross, if they are giving me the correct response, that's where they should see it. It is as precise and as quantifiable as any other technique you use.

So at the beginning I will settle for any part of the answer, just getting the two eyes working, but before I am through, I want the precision that is available. In general, the exotrope, when he is functioning in this type of instrument, will report quite accurately were he sees it. We break this down in the office into three aspects. One is spatial localization, the actual apparent localization of the target. Another is SILO. By simple laws of geometric projection when the target appears closer it should appear smaller and when it appears farther it should appear larger, The third aspect we look for is parallax. As the patient moves, the target should appear to move; when the instrument is set in base out disparity, a crossed disparity, the movement should follow the patient. If he moves to the right so should the target; if he squats it should go down, etc. If he moves back the target should appear farther from the screen, etc. although not at the same rate he is moving. When the targets are set for base in or uncrossed disparity, the parallax movement is opposite to the patient's movement. This is the same parallax phenomenon that you use in locating an opacity in ophthalmoscopy.

We look for virtuosity in giving us responses to this. How do we check the patient's responses? We can get part of the information from conversation. That isn't sufficient. We want actual localization and size judgments, and the only way we can identify that is to set real objects in the terrain so that they can give you landmarks. We have strings hanging down from the ceiling , things hanging into the projection scene, or we may move an object such as a pole on a moveable stand into the scene so that they can so they can discuss the relationship between the real and projected objects. If the distance is such that it is feasible, we let them reach out with their hands, or give them a pointer. The key is to have the patient match the perception of the projected image to real life space.

In general, with exotropes this does not present any great problem. Usually the exotrope has good ability to respond to stereoscopic cues. He has been using them before so you don't run into an enormous language or communication problems. He is habituated to responding to those types of cues, and in general it is not difficult to get good SILO and spatial localization. [As an aside – the same is not true when working with constant esotropes. They may have enormous difficulty matching their newly acquired spatial abilities in the controlled and contrived training situation with real world space. Often they cannot reconcile the cues available from binocular vision with their previous methods of mapping and functioning in the real world, including not having language constructs to explain what they are seeing. Or they may be able to describe an object apparently floating, but be incapable of reaching out to manually "touch" it. Constant esotropes may have deep fissures in their intersensory processing.]

Once having gotten this type of response, the training can proceed in several different directions, simultaneously. One would be a gradual introduction of more central targets. Another is the use of more detailed targets. Another would be an extension of the distances both inward and outward from the initial working distance. We might shift from projected anaglyph targets to projected vectograph targets which in general have more specific internal detail, or with overhead projector targets which are more detailed and central rather than just peripheral targets. When this can be maintained, we then go back over the sequence, and see if we can maintain the binocular functions in regard to alignment, stereopsis, spatial localization and parallax, with blur introduced whether in the form of lenses the patient wears or de-focusing of our target material.

During this time it is not uncommon to find that a change in the characteristic ocular alignment of the patient begins to take place. About this time in your training, the periodic exotropia should be appearing far less frequently. There should be periods of time when the patent is now straight eyed. At this time we may entertain the notion of going into closed instrument training so long as the patient can function in a straight posture. In other words, we put them into a stereoscope and let them work on AN series cards with stereopsis, or we may go into the Rotoscope with a stereoscopic target or the synoptophore with stereoscopic targets provided they can function in a straight ahead or ortho position. They may be able to hold alignment in the closed instrument for only a few minutes before diverging. WHEN THIS OCCURS, WE STOP THE PROCEDURE. We are not trying to make them aware of diplopia. I do not want to call attention to diplopia. I don't want them walking around fighting diplopia all the time. I want them posturing straight ahead. I will utilize closed instrument procedures only at an ortho setting, hoping to reinforce straight eyed ocular posture. This is easiest when stereo cards are used. As soon as the patient reaches his limit at any particular session, the activity is stopped for that day.

When this is more stable and we can get reasonably good work for reasonably long periods of time, we begin to work thru the sequence of cards backwards. We work with cards with less intense stereoscopic cues and finally we will work back towards the use of simultaneous perception materials in the Brock Series of Keystone cards toward BU l, which are just color cards, in an attempt to get luster, superimposition, or a picture in front of one eye end a color for luster in front of the other eye. This comes last. We are asking them to hold their eyes straight in the absence of stereopsis., because that is their problem. They don't bother holding the eyes straight when there is no particular reason for it. I want to train them hold eyes aligned under all circumstances.

About this time you can begin what I call posturing training, using a modification of the Brock Posture Box. You should become familiar with this modality. It is a great device and has a great application. Brock has had some very ingenuous ideas. He introduced the profession to the entire concept of working with projected anaglyphs and peripheral stimulation. Everyone has been working with color separation using red and green the anaglyph materials along with red and green filters. Brock had the insight to realize that if you used red and green filters with a red light and red print you would get better results, without the need for green or blue-green printing. Essentially, the technique makes use of projected red light which passes through the red filter but not the green filter, and a red target seen by reflected light which appears black through the green. Brock invented a device which is a red Plexiglas screen behind which there is a movable light, on top of which he puts red printed material. You put the anaglyphs on, one eye sees the light, the other eye sees the red printed material. You get no ghosts, you get no second images such as you do with the red and green printed material.

We use a variation of this. We draw a red ring (chalkboard work) We use a red light. and surround it with an annulus of red. Put a pair of red green filters on, the red filter transmits the light but doesn't permit the ring to be seen since the entire target looks red through the red filter. The green filter blocks out the light and transmits the annulus to be seen . In effect, one eye is seeing the light, the other eye is seeing the ring, and his job is to keep the light in the ring. We will start at the distance at which he can do it, then back up. the patient's task is to keep the light centered in the ring. We are training posture of the eyes, not fusion or stereopsis. and keep the light in the ring. This can be done very simply with a piece of cardboard with a hole in middle, a piece of red cellophane over the hole, a flashlight behind the hole and a target surrounding the hole drawn with a red pencil. With anaglyphs it provides a simple home training devices. The task is to keep the light in the middle as it is moved around at varying. distances.

In our office training, we do little or no base out or convergence training. For every bit of base out training we do, we do as much base in. We are interested in fusion ranges, quality of fusion, SILO, spatial localization, and ocular posture. We do extensive monocular training for accuracy of pursuits and saccades with some emphasis on insuring correct spatial interpretation of eye movements on saccades utilizing prism saccadic training. There is also emphasis on accommodative facility training. But there is no emphasis at all on developing convergence – it isn't necessary. You aren't going to get him to hold straight by building base out ductions.

There is one other thing in the training of the intermittent exotrope which is absolutely vital, and that is the use of lenses. If all you do is the training described you get pretty good results, but you won't get maximum results because there is a lens fitting approach with the divergent excess strabismic which has remarkable effectiveness. For those of you who are OEP oriented, you have all heard Skeff talk about the handling of exophoria with binocular plus. You have all heard also how far point exophoria can come about as a consequence of near point stress. The B2 syndrome in particular has a great deal in common with divergence excess. The infrequent instance where the exotropia begins after the child starts school is clearly predicted in the Skeffington model.

When the history indicates that the problem has been present since, let's say, one year of age, it becomes quite hard for me to accept the concept of a near point stress activity as being the instigating mechanism. Nonetheless, many years ago I noticed a parallel between the analytical measurements that I was getting on these youngsters and the B syndrome of OEP. This occurred almost without exception. At some point in the training program, the analytical findings show near point esophoria and prescribable plus. This seems to coincide with reports of the distance exotropia occurring very infrequently. It also seems that the emergence of this measurement of near esophoria is not a gradual event, but rather a sudden step function. We have seen this so often that my partner and I will say: "Jimmy popped today". A significant near esophoria is measured that was never noted previously. The phoria may be as high as 8 to 10 prism diopters. It will move lower in a week or so and seem to stabilize at a lower amount of esophoria accompanied by blur findings indicating need for a near add. It will swing back down a bit and stabilize at a lower amount of esophoria. At that point we prescribe near point plus in bifocal form. Usually, the near add is fairly low, in the order of +1.00 D. Most of the exospores leave the office wearing Plano adds. While, the OPEN premise that the B case is a response to near activities does not seem to be the basis for early onset intermittent divergent strabismus, once this stage of near esophoria appears, the patient behaves just like the OEP B case and that model places the near eso as the potential precursor of far point exophoria or exotropia.

Let me explain this using a different vocabulary. Let's think about the possible significance of the use of a plus add for near on these previously exotropic patients. This is very explainable in terms of continuing therapy on the basis of the ACA concept. When I finally get this individual to the point where he is functioning straight eyed almost of the time, with the deviation very infrequent except under extreme fatigue, what might be the benefit of a near add? I now have a person who shows me pretty solid binocular integration. and I dismiss them with a plano add to be used for school and reading and writing activities. The amount of plus is very modest: +.75 to +1.25 in most cases What is the effect of putting plus on at this time? The lens is dictated on the basis of better balance in near point findings. In effect, in putting plus lens on this individual for their reading activities, I am asking them to relatively converge more than they accommodate when doing near activities. I effectively put them into a continuing training program. When they look up from near to far, this habituated response is exactly what I would like them to be doing in order to control the tendency to deviate outward at distance fixation.

At the conclusion of active training, most patients are essentially free of a deviation. the cosmetic problem is solved, they are free of symptoms, and functioning quite well in all areas. It may take a prolonged cover test to fully dissociate them, but a high exophoria can still be detected. Sometimes we have to do the cover test for quite a long time before they will break. They will hold their eye posture at ortho against your cover test, but sooner or later you can get it. Those who follow through and continue to use their near adds show a different pattern. On subsequent examination, over a number of years, the far point exophoria gradually reduces. I have a number of youngsters who, when we dismiss them will still measure 22 exo at distance; they will come back in a year and measure 18, a year later 14 and gradually over a period of 5-7 years they will move down to a point where you can no longer detect a far point phoria. Some who have stopped wearing their lenses have shown regression and even return of some intermittent tropia. We put them back into the lenses and without further active training, the phoria moves back down while the turn disappears. There seems to be a distinct relationship between the continued use of plus and the ultimate modification of the far point exophoria.

The lens I am talking about is one that is very definitely prescribable from the measurements. The OEP analysis clearly calls for the near add and the add balances PRA, NRA, and near prism vergence blur points when utilizing graphical analysis. Aside from any immediate benefit that might be derived from prescribing such an add in terms of the patient comfort or efficiency, the prescription is a powerful tool for maintaining long term stability and control over the divergence excess strabismus. Regression is rare among those who continue use of their near add prescription.

Management of Divergence Excess Intermittent Exotropia

Nathan Flax, O.D.
J Behav Optom 1996;7(3):66, 72-3

Abstract

A method of treating divergence excess intermittent exotropia which differs from standard orthoptics is presented. Training is not done at the objective angle; ARC is ignored; diplopia awareness is not cultivated; stereoscopic targets are introduced before flat fusion or simultaneous perception targets; little emphasis is placed on developing base-out prism vergence ranges; monocular skills and accommodative facility are developed; and plus adds are utilized. The rationale for this approach is developed.

Key Words

exotropia, divergence excess, strabismus, orthoptics, vision therapy

For more than 30 years, I have been treating divergence excess intermittent exotropia in a highly successful way which produces excellent long-term control.[1,2] This approach differs from other methods in the following ways:

1. No attempt is made to make the patient aware of diplopia.
2. Training is not done at the angle of squint.
3. Anomalous retinal correspondence (ARC) is ignored.
4. Stereoscopic targets are utilized first, followed by second degree targets. Simultaneous perception targets are utilized last.
5. Relatively little emphasis is placed on increasing base-out prism vergence ability.
6. Monocular skills and accommodative facility are emphasized.
7. Near plus in bifocal form is utilized for long-term control.

The goal of my treatment is to achieve alignment without conscious effort by developing a postural vergence set for straight eyes. A basic premise of my approach is that tonic vergence, rather than fusional vergence to avoid diplopia, is the primary mechanism by which normal individuals maintain straight eyes. This differs from standard orthoptic methods which emphasize diplopia awareness and development of fusional vergence to overcome latent strabismus.[3,4] Diplopia awareness has little place in normal seeing. While it can be used as a tool to trigger fusion, this is not natural. Brock stated: "If the norm for any behavioral characteristic is determined by its frequency of occurrence, then it must be conceded that the awareness of physiologic diplopia is an entirely abnormal experience: . . . The fact that you can 'teach' them to see double in a matter of minutes does not alter this fact."[5]

Intermittent exotropes of the divergence excess type usually can demonstrate fusion, including high level stereopsis before therapy is initiated. Their binocular vision is closer to that of normals than to constant strabismics since they can demonstrate sensory fusion and bifoveal motor alignment at the same time, a condition that constant strabismics cannot meet. Their problem is not lack of sensory fusion, but rather an inability to maintain alignment on a consistent basis. My approach emphasizes reinforcement of straight eye posture rather than elimination of suppression or ARC when the eyes are turned. Suppression and ARC are considered to be adaptations that will fade when they are no longer useful to the patient. If the turn is intermittent, it is not even necessary to test for ARC. A guiding principle is that the sensory status when deviated becomes moot if the deviation itself is eliminated by developing tonic postural vergence. Training at the angle of turn is avoided and the problem of ARC is finessed. If present, ARC disappears as the patient gains motor control over the deviation.

My training regimen reverses the usual order of presentation of binocular stimuli. The usual schema of classifying fusion stimuli as first degree simultaneous binocular awareness, second degree flat fusion, and third degree stereopsis implies a hierarchical relationship which does not exist in the real world. Simultaneous awareness of dissimilar foveally viewed targets is not encountered under normal circumstances. It can occur only if the patient is strabismic or if a carefully structured artificial environment is created by use of a stereoscope, vectographs, anaglyphs, or a distorting device such as a Maddox rod. First degree binocular awareness is not likely to be a stage in the development of normal binocular vision. Flat fusion is also rarely encountered in the real world. There are almost no conditions in which the two eyes do not receive disparity cues. Even when looking at a flat page or CRT screen, the overall scene contains stereoscopic cues. Almost all natural stimulus conditions are essentially stereoscopic. It requires special manipulation of the visual inputs to achieve flat fusion.

Intermittent exotropes are unconsciously selective in the manner in which they utilize binocular vision, aligning the eyes when binocular cues are useful and allowing an eye to deviate when there is little benefit from binocular vision. The turn often occurs when "daydreaming." Parents of young children note that the child's eyes straighten whenever there is attention to the task at hand. For those patients whose turn is present at near as well as at distance, the push-up near point of convergence may be receded. However, when the same target is utilized with instructions to localize it (as in the stick in straw test), convergence improves. These patients find it easiest to fuse stereoscopic targets. They find it more difficult to fuse and maintain alignment when there is no intrinsic benefit to binocular vision. This is the reason for my reversal of the standard order of presentation of stimuli. I begin with stereoscopic targets and gradually introduce second degree and finally simultaneous perception targets. The goal of treatment is to have the patient maintain straight eyes even when stereopsis is not useful or available.

Since the goal of treatment is to develop a postural set for straight eyes, no activities are done which would reward or reinforce the patient when the eyes are in the deviated position. Training is not done at the angle of turn. Binocular activities are introduced at the ortho setting utilizing stereoscopic targets since these are more likely to permit the patient to hold alignment. Straight eye posture is rewarded and the stimuli are gradually modified from stereoscopic to second degree to simultaneous perception with continual emphasis on holding posture. When the patient cannot hold alignment, the activity is modified by providing a stronger stimulus to fusion rather than calling attention to diplopia. Quality of fusion is emphasized, including attention to spatial localization and SILO when using vectographic and anaglyphic targets. Peripheral stereopsis using projected targets is the usual starting point of binocular treatment. Most of the early binocular training does not involve closed stereoscope or amblyoscope procedures because the patient usually cannot succeed in fusing at ortho in these instruments. Closed instrument tasks are introduced when the patient can perform at ortho. Third degree targets are used initially and then followed by second degree and finally first degree targets.

It is generally not necessary to emphasize development of base-out vergence ranges since fusional convergence tends to restore spontaneously as the patient responds to the treatment approach. The notion of increasing fusional convergence assumes that the fundamental problem is structural exophoria. My approach is based on a different premise regarding the etiology of divergence excess. Early in my career I noted inconsistencies in the behavior of many divergence excess patients which could not be reconciled with a standard graphical analysis model of binocular vision. The positive relative accommodation-negative relative accommodation (PRA-NRA) relationship often was at variance with what might be expected for an exophore, with the negative relative amplitude high and the positive relative amplitude low. Some showed near esophoria which was not consistent with the distance deviation. During treatment, the near lateral phoria of some patients changed abruptly in the direction of esophoria despite the fact that the treatment had not been heavily involved with development of near convergence. The blur, break, and recovery of the prism vergence measurements were not always consistent, nor did they respond to treatment in the same way.

These behaviors are not readily explained by graphical analysis, but they are by the OEP-Skeffington model.[6] The B-case type of Skeffington and divergence excess bear striking similarities.[7] The OEP model predicts development of far-point exophoria as a response to an inability to sustain attention at near. At risk of oversimplification, the scenario is briefly as follows: The effort needed to function at demanding near tasks creates a drive to converge at a plane closer than accommodation. The patient becomes esophoric at near and must inhibit fusional convergence to maintain single vision. The habituated behavioral pattern of inhibition of convergence (or active divergence relative to accommodation) is an appropriate compensation to permit performance at near. This behavior pattern is then carried over to distance activities resulting in myopia or divergence excess. Such a patient would show near esophoria, reduced accommodative facility, a low PRA, and high NRA. The near base-out vergence finding would show a high blur since base-out prism permits convergence at a closer plane than accommodation. Once the break point has been reached, the recovery to fusion measurement would be low since the patient has been inhibiting fusional convergence. Each component of the prism vergence measurements has a different basis in this model and need not co-vary.

Skeffington[6] explains this sequence of adaptive behaviors as a response to the intense near demands of our society. Utilization of plus lenses at near satisfies the drive to converge closer than accommodate and permits the patient to maintain clear, single binocular vision without developing compensatory behaviors which then become inappropriate at distance. Application of near plus is expected to impact distance measurements by inhibiting the development of far point exophoria and/or myopia. Divergence excess strabismus usually begins long before school age and could not be due to the social demands of our culture in most cases. An alternative possibility is that a slightly high ACA ratio produces excessive accommodative convergence, requiring the patient to utilize fusional divergence at near to maintain single vision, setting a scenario similar to that postulated by Skeffington. Regardless of etiology, the measurement profile of the divergence excess patient is quite similar to that of the OEP B case. This similarity led me to treat divergence excess patients as if they were in fact OEP B cases. This has been my strategy for long-term management of these patients.

Most patients with divergence excess whom I have encountered demonstrate poor oculomotor control on a monocular basis and accommodative inefficiency along with their binocular problem, still further resembling the OEP B type case. These skills are trained along with fusion. Divergence excess patients treated in this manner follow the pattern predicted by the Skeffington model. Almost invariably, the measurements resemble a B case as alignment is achieved. At this point a near add is called for based upon OEP precepts; the near phoria is eso and the add normalizes both near prism vergence blur findings and the PRA-NRA relationship. The divergence prism vergence measures may actually be lower than the convergence range. Vergence range extension training may be undertaken at this juncture, but the purpose is to normalize binocular function rather than to develop compensation to overcome exophoria. Both divergence and convergence are developed along with voluntary convergence on non-fusible simultaneous perception targets. Near plus is prescribed in bifocal form to satisfy the drive to center (converge) closer than the plane of identification (accommodation). This has a salutary effect on the long-term stability of the condition. With the need to adapt at near relieved, far point exophoria (which was induced by the near adaptation) often reduces. Those patients who continue to utilize their reading lenses after formal training is completed often show gradual reduction of far exophoria over a period of years.

This approach to treating intermittent strabismus of the divergence excess type has been very successful. Patients respond rapidly and show little or no regression after completion of formal training. In addition to resolution of the cosmetic problem, improvement in scholastic and/or athletic performance is almost invariably reported.

References

1. *Flax N. The optometric treatment of intermittent divergent strabismus. Eastern Seaboard Vision Training Conference, Washington. DC. 1963; transcript by Caryl Croissant, Morro Bay, CA.*

2. *Flax N. San Jose Vision Training Seminar. 1968, San Jose, CA; transcript by Caryl Croissant. Morro Bay, CA.*

3. *Caloroso EE, Rouse MW. Clinical Management of Strabismus. Butterworth-Heinemann, 1993:26.*

4. *Rosner J, Rosner J. Pediatric Optometry, 2nd Ed. Butterworths, 1990:508-9.*

5. *Brock FW. Visual training-part III, Optom Wkly 1959 Jan 1:11.*

6. *Skeffington AM. Optometric Extension Program Continuing Education Courses. Optom Ext Prog; 1928-1974.*

7 *Birnbaum MR. Optometric Management of Nearpoint Vision Disorders. Butterworth-Heinemann.1993:65.*

AMBLYOPIA

The three articles in this section pretty much summarize my approach to amblyopia. I wrote about pleoptics in 1961. This was heralded by ophthalmology in this country as a totally new way to treat amblyopia. I viewed it as development of more sophisticated instrumentation to accomplish things that optometrists had been doing for a long time. At that time, it was my feeling that European ophthalmology was far more interested in function than American ophthalmology. I suspect that this may still be so. The Visuoscope or its variants became part of my practice, as did the use of the Coordinator based upon the Haidinger Brush phenomenon. I purchased a Euthoscope but found it unusable without dilation (not available to me at that time). I suspect that it would have been of little use for me even with dilation. The instrument was a large, heavy, unwieldy ophthalmoscope. Having small hands, I could not manipulate the several switches while aiming the device.

I have always avoided prolonged occlusion. Short term occlusion with specific, directed activities works very well. Nor did I necessarily utilize full refractive correction as an initial step in treatment. It is difficult to obtain consistent or reliable responses when refracting an amblyopic eye. Beginning fixation training before deciding on a refractive correction often has the salutary effect of improving the patient's ability to detect and respond to finer discriminations. Sometimes the refraction begins to "normalize" once treatment has begun. Just be sure to use target materials within the patient's capability. A small light can be accurately fixated with almost any ametropia.

The prime reason for avoiding prolonged occlusion is based upon empathy for the patient. Bear in mind that functional amblyopia does not bother patients in daily activities. They may be less efficient because of poor binocular function, but the lack of clear central vision in the amblyopic eye does not adversely influence performance in tasks of daily living so long as both eyes are open. I have seen instances where the treatment was worse than the disease in terms of its impact on the behavior of the child.

Three papers follow.

Pleoptics and Functional Optometry

Nathan Flax, O.D., FAAO
Opt J Rev Opt 1961;48(17):27-30

Pleoptics refers to the theories, training procedures and devices developed by European ophthalmologists to treat amblyopia. It has been described as the active treatment of functional amblyopia. It embraces two slightly different approaches and a variety of devices such as the Visuscope, Euthyscope, Pleoptophor, Coordinator, Space Coordinator, Localizer, Corrector, and Separation Trainer.

The basic approaches are the products of Prof. Cuppers and Prof. Bangarter. Both techniques make use of after-images, although in slightly different fashions. Cuppers uses the entoptic phenomenon of Haidinger Brushes to provide a clue to direct fixation. Bangarter uses kinesthetic, tactile, and auditory reinforcement to train direct fixation. While based upon slightly different theories, there is a great deal of similarity in the two methods and hence they have come to be grouped together under the heading of pleoptics. This mode of amblyopia therapy now occupies much attention in ophthalmologic-orthoptic technician circles. It is being presented as the "newest" approach in vision training and is responsible for a rather startling upsurge of interest on the part of medicine in functional aspects of vision.

Dynamics of the Approach

It will be the purpose of this paper to briefly describe pleoptic theory and practice and to properly relate this therapy to the body of long-standing optometric thinking. No attempt will be made to quantifiably evaluate results of pleoptic therapy. Rather, the attempt will be made to indicate the dynamics of the approach in a way of which its proponents are apparently, as yet, unaware. By so doing, I hope that the following conclusions will be established:

(1)   Pleoptics is essentially a re-affirmation of the optometric concepts of functional vision.

(2)   Several quite valuable new diagnostic and training tools have emerged from this medical interest in amblyopia therapy.

(3)   Most of the pleoptic approaches involve refinement of optometric vision training techniques.

Thoughts on amblyopia

Before proceeding to pleoptics per se, it might be well to introduce some thoughts on amblyopia. Writing in the *American Orthoptic Journal* (Volume 10, 1960), Gunter K. von Noorden elaborates on the functional aspects of strabismus amblyopia. He differentiates between the amblyopia of pathology, the amblyopia of disuse, and the amblyopia of active inhibition. These latter two classifications are quite interesting. He points out that strabismus amblyopia should not be labeled ex anopsia since that term implies a passive condition of disuse. Rather, von Noorden feels that:

"The impairment is the result of long-lasting active inhibition of the macular function of form vision in the course of an adaptive mechanism, to avoid diplopia or confusion. The various theories regarding the origin and seat of this functional defect were discussed at length before this group three years ago. It may suffice to state that the seat is most likely in the visual cortex, and that the inhibition is selective in nature, inasmuch as certain basic visual functions, such as light sense, flicker fusion frequency, and visual acuity as measured with objective methods are less disturbed than the subjectively measured visual acuity, or are entirely normal."

This concept of purposeful adaptation is certainly consistent with optometric philosophy wherein the intactness of total organismic response is maintained at the expense of constriction of operational ranges and even at the price of ablating part of the monocular circuiting. This type of response to stress would be made in the area most susceptible. Hence, it is not surprising that the basic visual functions such as light sense, flicker fusion frequency, and objective visual acuity are relatively undisturbed. No adaptive need would be satisfied by disturbances of these functions. Inhibition of central form vision does permit more effective over-all operation.

A strong statement for functional optometric thinking is also contained in von Noorden's remark: "Under conditions in which the function of visual acuity plays a minor role (for example, in the dark), this inhibition becomes pointless and the amblyopic eye resembles the normal eye."

Valuable diagnostic tools

At this point it might be appropriate to describe the first of the valuable diagnostic tools to come out of the recognition of the adaptive nature of amblyopia. While this technique is not, strictly speaking, part of pleoptic technique, it is quite appropriate to our discussion. Again, the quotation is from von Noorden:

> *As was stated, recent work has shown that functions other than form vision are less disturbed in the amblyopic eye, or may even remain intact under certain conditions. Wald and Burian have demonstrated that the threshold of light recognition is essentially normal in the dark adapted amblyopic eye. Unsteady and jerky fixation is present in amblyopic eyes under conditions of ordinary lighting. This was shown by Mackensen with an electro-ophthalmographic method and was confirmed by us.*
>
> *But we were also able to demonstrate that in many amblyopic eyes complete recovery of the unsteady fixation behavior occurred as soon as these eyes were dark adapted. It was also found that no recovery occurred under dark adaptation in patients with organic amblyopia. The extraordinary capacities of the amblyopic eye under scotopic conditions induced us to measure visual acuity with the use of filters and at various levels of illumination. Using a neutral density filter with which the visual acuity of a normal eye was reduced to about one half, only little reduction, no change, or even improvement of visual acuity was noted when the filter was held before the amblyopic eye. However, when the same test was employed in eyes with anatomical damage to the macula, visual acuity was reduced to almost grotesque readings.*
>
> *The diagnostic importance of these findings is obvious. A determination of the visual acuity at various increasing levels of illumination revealed, furthermore, that the amblyopic eye behaved exactly like the normal control eye at low illuminations. In fact, it showed even relative improvement over the sound eye in several instances.*

Thus far amblyopia would seem to be involved solely with the identification process. Examination of the Cuppers and Bangarter approaches will reveal how adaptation in the centering mechanism can also give rise to amblyopia. It has long been known clinically that amblyopic patients frequently do better when single, isolated Snellen letters or other test types are presented, than when asked to read an entire line. In pleoptic literature this single letter acuity is called "angular" acuity to differentiate it from line acuity which is called "cortical" acuity. The discrepancy in acuity measurements is explained as a function of "crowding" or "separation difficulty."

Monocular diplopia

Cuppers explains this "separation difficulty" as being due to monocular diplopia in the amblyopic eye which is eccentrically fixating. When a line of letters is presented, there is superimposition of different letters and consequent confusion. When single letters, or a vertical row of letters are viewed, this lateral diplopia does not create confusion and hence the acuity is affected much less. The basis of this monocular diplopia is improper egocentric localization ability in the amblyopic eye. This is said to be a result of (and not the cause of) adaptation to a binocular problem. According to pleoptic concepts, the turned eye adopts a new subjective "straight ahead" localization using an eccentric point as its zero position as an adaptation to the binocular misalignment. This new subjective direction is then carried into the monocular act, resulting in eccentric fixation. Hence, monocular eccentric fixation and anomalous retinal correspondence may be considered as related phenomena. To again quote von Noorden on Cuppers theory: "Eccentric fixation occurs, so to speak, as the terminal process, of which anomalous correspondence is an intermediate step."

Under testing situations there may be a reawakening of the original spatial value of fovea as the zero position, giving rise to monocular diplopia. This would be quite similar to the binocular triplopia which can frequently be demonstrated in cases of anomalous retinal correspondence.

While not stated in these terms, the foregoing analysis can comfortably be described as an adaptive shift in the centering process to permit total functioning, even at the expense of ignoring or modifying part of one monocular input circuit. It is most interesting to note the emphasis on adaptive function and the realization that clinical problems may be the results of function as well as organic structure.

The measuring ophthalmoscope

With these conceptual thoughts in mind, the chief diagnostic tool of pleoptics (in addition to the previously mentioned filter tests and differentiation between line and single letter acuity) is a measuring ophthalmoscope known as a Visuscope. This device permits projection of a fixation target and measuring concentric circles (or a grid) onto the patient's retina. The optics of the system permit both patient and examiner to view the targets simultaneously. Thus, it is possible to determine exactly which retinal point is being used for subjective "straight ahead" by the patient. Wisely, it is concluded that if the patient consistently picks the same extra-foveal point for his fixation point, then occlusion of the better eye is contra-indicated. This type of occlusion will tend to embed a faulty pattern rather than eliminate it. In cases of unstable or wandering fixation, standard occlusion therapy might be beneficial.

More significant to our discussion is the recommendation to occlude the *amblyopic* eye in cases of steady eccentric fixation. The obvious attempt here is to disembed by removing the stressor agent (namely, the need to match egocentric localization in two circuits). This type of therapy is not new to optometry. Although the method is not new or radical to functional optometry, the instrument itself represents a major advance in diagnostic equipment. Unfortunately, the corneal reflex and other tests are crude when one considers that we are at times dealing with angles of eccentricity of a fraction of a degree. Here, even in optometric vision training, the possibility of embedding rather than eliminating a faulty monocular pattern exists. The Visuscope provides an excellent method of checking the accuracy of the mechanical aspects of the centering process.

Use of after-images

The training techniques of pleoptics are all designed to permit the patient to use the fovea as his reference point for directionality. Cuppers makes use of after-images with the Euthyscope, which is another modified ophthalmoscope. This instrument is designed so that the operator can illuminate the patient's retina peripherally, while shielding the macula area. By use of high intensity illumination, a doughnut-shaped after image can be created, with the fovea as its center. By flashing, a negative after-image is created so that the patient is aware of a bright spot surrounded by darkness in his monocular field of view. He is asked to consciously attempt to aim this bright spot where he is looking.

This is a rather ingenious method of providing an information control circuit to the patient to permit more accurate centering. This type of approach has been used optometrically to develop normal retinal correspondence. Its use in the monocular situation represents an advance which might have considerable value in non-strabismic and non-amblyopic optometric vision training.

The ring-shaped after image is also designed to temporarily raise the light threshold of the surrounding retina, thereby giving physiologic superiority to the macular area over the normally used eccentric fixation area. Bangarter makes much use of this principle in his Pleoptophor. This is an elaborate instrument which permits initial dazzling of the peripheral retina with bright light and then later accurately aimed stimulation of the fovea itself with flashing light. In principle this is not dissimilar to some of the older optometric amblyopia training utilizing flashing and high intensity stimulation. The technique refinements are, however, major steps forward.

Both Cuppers and Bangarter rely heavily on reestablishment of accurate foveal fixation. Cuppers utilizes the projected afterimage and also makes use of Haidinger Brushes. This is an entoptic phenomenon whereby a rotating Polaroid filter produces a brush-like appearance centered around the projection of the anatomical fovea. He uses an instrument called the Coordinator (and modifications such as the Space Coordinator and Coordinator combined with a synoptophore) to produce the Haidinger Brush pattern. This provides another means of reference to the patient attempting to realign subjective visual direction with anatomical straight-ahead. While not new, the clinical utilization of this aspect of vision is rather ingenious and indicative of a growing willingness on the part of ophthalmology to explore into functional aspects of vision.

A familiar approach

Professor Bangarter's approach to development of proper egocentric localization in amblyopic eyes is quite familiar to optometry. He makes much use of other sense modalities to orient visual localization. With a series of devices not at all dissimilar to those described frequently by William Smith in the optometric literature, he makes use of hand-eye and auditory-visual coordination to obtain accurate eye fixation.

The Localizor and Corrector, and variations thereof, are instruments which permit either tactile or auditory reinforcement for training accuracy of eye fixation. Much has been done for many years and still is being done in this regard in standard optometric vision training. Here, again, the possibilities of these devices in non-amblyopic patients should be investigated. They perhaps offer a method of refinement of optometric application certainly not considered by their originators.

Still another training device utilized by Bangarter is his Separation Trainer. This is a device which permits varying the separation between letters, as the patient views them on a screen with intermittent illumination. As the patient can resolve the letters, they are brought closer together or the patient is moved further from the screen. Optometrically, this form of training, with slight variation, is known as Updegrave training and is frequently an integral part of vision training programs.

Summary

In summary, this paper has attempted to outline pleoptic theory, instrumentation, and technique. The strong parallel between the underlying dynamics of pleoptics and functional optometry has been pointed out. Similarities between standard optometric vision training and the "new" pleoptics have been shown. The use of pleoptic theory as a defense (if such is necessary) for optometric philosophy has also been indicated. Real advances in instrumentation, new diagnostic procedures, and improvement upon existing training techniques have been described. Pleoptics is unlikely to become a panacea. Rather, it is more apt to find its rightful place in the spectrum of visual diagnostic and therapeutic procedures. Much of it is not really new, but rather revitalized. Certainly, the great ophthalmological interest in this facet of vision training can be interpreted as a shift in medical orientation toward the functional concepts so long espoused by optometry.

Some Thoughts on the Clinical Management of Amblyopia

Nathan Flax, O.D.
State College of Optometry, State University of New York, New York, New York
Am J Optom 1983;60(6):450-3

Abstract
Brief periods of ocular occlusion, coupled with careful reinforcement of the desired behavior, are frequently more effective than prolonged direct occlusion in the treatment of amblyopia.

Key Words
amblyopia treatment, part-time occlusion

Traditionally, prolonged direct occlusion of the preferred eye has been the mainstay of amblyopia therapy. In recent years there has been reassessment of this procedure, generally motivated by fear of development of occlusion amblyopia in the previously normal eye due to deprivation of light and form vision during the early critical stage of vision development[1] Among many optometrists seriously engaged in strabismus and amblyopia therapy, however, constant occlusion has been largely replaced by part-time occlusion for other reasons, apart from the fear of occlusion amblyopia. These reasons are: to avoid an increase in the overt angle of strabismus,[2] humane considerations involving the burden placed on a deeply amblyopic subject by denying use of the good eye in a competitive school environment, and development of effective techniques which permit successful results using intermittent occlusion and specific training procedures.

The important aspects of amblyopia treatment can be discussed in terms of five factors, four of which have presented by previous participants in this symposium. The factors to be considered are:

1. Oculomotor control and fixation
2. Spatial perception
3. Accommodative efficiency
4. Binocular function
5. Refractive correction.

Although the above components are not usually specifically identified as such, analysis of optometric therapy procedures generally discloses that one or more of the cited factors is a critical element in successful treatment. The key to success lies in structuring activities to develop each of the first four factors, and in proper use of refractive correction.

Amblyopes are characteristically poor at oculomotor control and fixation. Instead of just asking the child to wander around with the better eye covered in the hope that fixation will improve, it is far more effective to set up appropriate feedback and to work intensively for brief periods of time. At the crudest level, when fixation is very erratic, having the parent observe the corneal light reflex as the child attempts to fixate a muscle light while offering verbal reinforcement when the eye is close to being centered on the target can be effective. As fixation accuracy develops, more specific and refined visual feedback can be supplied using entopic phenomena such as the Haidinger brush or Maxwell's spot. Foveally placed afterimages can also be used to provide visual feedback to the patient regarding the accuracy of ocular fixation. Tracking a moving target can improve accuracy of dynamic aspects of oculomotor control. A series of specifically guided training sessions during the course of the day, each for a few minutes at a time but with close supervision and proper feedback and reinforcement, can produce as much favorable change as a full day of simple occlusion with no appropriate conditioning applied. In one study, use of twice-weekly training more than tripled the speed of response to occlusion therapy.[3]

In addition to reduced visual acuity, amblyopes frequently demonstrate impaired spatial perception. They have difficulty localizing objects with the amblyopic eye and often demonstrate a greater functional handicap than might be anticipated on the basis of their visual acuity. An amblyope with 20/200 acuity behaves differently than does an uncorrected myope or other ametrope with the same visual acuity. Often amblyopes show difficulty pointing to or reaching for objects well above their resolution threshold. Their ability to navigate using primarily visual information seems impaired. It is probable that the visual acuity improvements that result from occlusion derive from development of more normal spatial monocular perception, for this is the factor that is best addressed by simple total occlusion for long periods of time. At the outset of occlusion, the patient with deep amblyopia is typically handicapped in his or her normal environment. Characteristically, the ability to navigate, reach, touch, and orient improves with occlusion time, followed later by visual acuity improvement. It is possible, however, to produce these changes fairly rapidly by careful structuring of training activities done during brief periods of patching without need for long-term activities. Aiming, orienting, touching, and visually guided movement procedures with appropriate opportunity to monitor error are easily set up and can be extremely effective in amblyopia therapy. At a more refined level, pleoptic techniques combine spatial perception and fixation training. Similar procedures have been described for many years in the optometric literature.[4]

Another functional deficiency demonstrated by amblyopes is impaired accommodative ability. Whether this is secondary to fixation inaccuracy, eccentric fixation, or a deficiency in its own right, improvement in accommodative response seems to parallel the visual acuity improvement. For this reason, accommodative facility training is an effective tool in successful amblyopia therapy, and is another factor which is best treated in a systematic, controlled fashion. While the accommodative amplitude measured by bringing the target close to the patient may be lower in the amblyopic eye than in the fellow eye, there may be a still greater discrepancy between the two eyes when accommodation is measured by introduction of concave lenses with the target held at a fixed distance. In the absence of proximal cues, amblyopes seem to have difficulty responding to the blur induced by change in the vergence of light entering the eye. The amplitude measured by concave lenses may show a more severe reduction relative to the sound eye than the amplitude measured by a push-up technique. Treatment techniques which emphasize response to lens-induced vergence seem more effective than procedures which use target distance to generate the accommodative stimulus.

Amblyopes characteristically show reduced binocular function. If not overtly strabismic, they generally demonstrate suppression, reduced stereopsis, or both. An important aspect of amblyopia therapy is, therefore, development of fusion with the hope of ultimate bifoveal fixation and high level binocular integration. This is not to be interpreted as meaning that there must be amblyopia in the presence of strabismus. Patients with spontaneous alternation can and do show excellent visual acuity. Amblyopia is generally related to constant unilateral strabismus or to anisometropia. The key factor in the development of suppression amblyopia is persistent suppression of the fovea of the amblyopic eye to avoid confusion. (Suppression to avoid diplopia is not the key factor in development of amblyopia because this involves a peripheral locus in the deviating eye). In the case of a unilateral strabismic with normal retinal correspondence, the object imaged on the fovea of the deviated eye is referred to the same place in space and confused with the object of regard imaged on the foveal of the fixing eye. In the case of a non-strabismic with uncorrected anisometropia, the confusion is between a clear image seen by the less ametropic eye and the blurred image of the ametropic eye, both of which are referred to the same place in space. In either situation, suppression in the fovea of the amblyopic eye develops to avoid such confusion.

The key to binocular treatment to improve amblyopia lies in the elimination of the need to suppress. This can only be achieved with proper refractive correction, alignment of the eyes, and development of binocular integrative capacity. In the absence of any one of these factors, amblyopia therapy cannot have permanence (except in the situation where the patient develops alternating strabismus in place of fusion). Given these constraints, it should be noted that strabismus surgery is rarely an effective treatment for amblyopia. Reduction in angle of deviation cannot be expected to have any impact on amblyopia unless the surgery produces precise bifoveal fixation in all directions of gaze and the patient spontaneously demonstrates cessation of suppression and full binocular integration. Merely reducing the deviation to cosmetically acceptable limits cannot be expected to cure or even reduce amblyopia. This is not generally well understood. Reports of amblyopia treated surgically must be very carefully assessed, for while this may on occasion be possible, the probabilities are very low. Orthoptic treatment, on the other hand, can often be effective in reducing amblyopia by elimination of suppression and development of binocular integration.

The last factor in the therapy of amblyopia that I would like to discuss is refractive correction. This presents significant management problems for the clinician. On one hand, it is desirable to provide optimum imagery for each eye in early infancy. In theory this might eliminate the confusion of anisometropia and thus abort the amblyopia process. But countering this approach are two other considerations. Refractive measurements are highly unstable in early infancy (the very period with which there is greatest concern) and, additionally, anisometropic correction carries the risk of interfering with binocular function by creating unequal retinal image sizes or difficulty with variable prismatic effects in different directions of gaze. The presently available diagnostics to properly assess the optical impact of anisometropic correction are not applicable to infants. Perhaps measurement of all refractive components including axial length, intraocular component spacing, lens power in vivo, in addition to refractive error, might permit better prediction, but such is not yet the state of the art. Early use of contact lenses is sometimes offered as an approach, but it must be borne in mind that size effects of contact lenses and spectacles are not always predictable.

The clinician must therefore still deal with the difficult problem of management of refractive correction without stable data or complete predictability of the influence of the lens correction on binocular function. This author sometimes makes use of temporary correction for specific training activities on a part-time basis so as to achieve the benefits of optical correction during the period of time of specific therapy directed toward improvement of fixation, spatial orientation on a monocular basis, and development of accommodative facility, while at the same time avoiding the possibility of adversely influencing binocular development. This is a particularly useful approach with very high anisometropia. Spectacles can be used just during the periods of active monocular treatment of the amblyopic eye, permitting improvement in three of the four previously discussed factors. If there is a positive response, then the patient becomes better able to participate at binocular testing, enabling a more intelligent decision as to preferred optical management during the attempts at binocular development. This is a more easily controlled approach than beginning with a contact lens for the highly myopic eye not knowing what to predict as an outcome.

The therapeutic approaches that are successful in treating amblyopia are those that are directed toward development of more accurate eye movement control, improvement in spatial perception, improvement in accommodative facility, and elimination of suppression with improvement of binocular integration, along with providing appropriate optical correction. Often all these therapeutic factors serve to potentiate one another. At other times, as indicated above in the description of a particular anisometropic condition, some may be antagonistic to one another. Under such conditions, clinical decisions may not be clear-cut. When it may not be possible to achieve full correction of amblyopia accompanied by completely normal bifoveal fusion, there is need for a trade-off between level of visual acuity and other aspects of vision function. This is particularly true in the case of intermittent strabismus with amblyopia, or low-angle strabismus with peripheral fusion where prolonged patching can improve acuity but leave the patient with a large-angle constant turn. Because the goal is to achieve binocular function as well as visual acuity improvement, it is necessary to use therapeutic approaches which do not achieve one objective at the price of the other.

Prolonged total occlusion, particularly where the amblyopia is deep, can have an enormous adverse effect of the overall performance and development of a youngster who is forced to compete at a major disadvantage in school and other situations. This author has seen children with significant secondary emotional and social problems resulting from dogmatic and insensitive application of relatively nonproductive total occlusion. The well-being of the child as a person was sacrificed for minimal gain in acuity of the amblyopic eye. One has to question whether the result was worth the price. The continued deprivation imposed by not letting a child use a good eye for long periods of time can have perhaps more serious overall consequences than the amblyopia itself. If total occlusion does not produce fairly rapid response it should be abandoned in favor of other strategies, particularly because periodic occlusion may actually be more effective than prolonged patching.[5]

In my practice, constant occlusion of the amblyopic eye to disrupt stable eccentric fixation and alternating occlusion to minimize the possibility of anomalous retinal correspondence developing in young constant squinters who cannot respond to sophisticated training procedures are about the only circumstances in which any degree of prolonged occlusion is used. In almost all other instances, short-term patching combined with highly controlled tasks involving eye movement, spatial perception, accommodation, and binocular interaction is sufficient to produce positive clinical responses.

The research results reported at this symposium serve both to support the clinical approaches that have been used over the years and also to point the way toward development of new and more effective techniques for the management of amblyopia. Isolation and specification of the underlying factors of amblyopia should lead the clinician-researcher team to more effective patient care.

Acknowledgement

I wish to thank Dr. K. Ciuffreda for his helpful comments.

References

1. Burian HM. Occlusion amblyopia and the development of eccentric fixation in occluded eyes. Am J Ophthalmol 1966;62:853-6.
2. Schapero M. Amblyopia. Philadelphia: Chilton, 1971;186-90.
3. Francois J, James M. Comparative study of amblyopic treatment. Am Orthopt J 1 955;5:61-4.
4. Smith WS. Clinical Orthoptic Procedures. 2nd ed. St Louis: CV Mosby, 1954;91-7.
5. Crewther DP, Crewther SG, Mitchell DE. The efficacy of brief periods of reverse occlusion in promoting recovery from the physiologic effects of monocular deprivation in kittens. Invest Ophthalmol Vis Sci 1981;21:357-62.

Common Sense Management of Amblyopia - Amblyopes Are People, Not Eyes

Nathan Flax, O.D.
J Opt Vis Dev 1995;26(2):53-6

Abstract
An approach that differs from the standard model of amblyopia treatment is presented. Alternatives to total occlusion, full refractive correction, and vigorous elimination of suppression can produce excellent results. The methods offered are less traumatic and less disruptive to the patient than standard therapy.

Key Words
amblyopia, occlusion, anisometropia, fusion, refractive correction

Standard therapy for amblyopia requires full refractive correction, intensive occlusion, and elimination of suppression. There are two reasons why this approach may not be the best way to proceed, even though improvement in acuity is often attained. First, other management strategies may be as effective as this approach, but have fewer adverse side effects. Second, standard therapy may be harmful to the patient despite improvement in visual acuity.

This latter consideration is often overlooked in well-meaning, zealous attempts to achieve acuity in an amblyopic eye, particularly when acuity is pursued aggressively with very young patients. Iatrogenic ally induced amblyopia in the formerly dominant eye is documented, and current good practice calls for careful monitoring and modification of occlusion strategies to minimize this possibility. The effects of occlusion on other aspects of early visual development such as eye-hand coordination and form perception have not been investigated and are rarely considered in management plans.

Amblyopic eyes are deficient in localization and spatial perception in addition to having reduced acuity. Forcing a child to function with the normally fixing eye patched is not a trivial procedure when viewed in terms of its potential impact on the overall behavior of the child. Intensive occlusion of patients with amblyopia can interfere with development of normal dexterity as well as academic and social skills. To develop empathy for the plight of the youngster wearing a patch, the reader is invited to spend a week or even a day with his or her preferred hand tied down. Frustration at writing can be enormous. Being forced to use a clumsy hand can cause reduced understanding of material presented at a lecture while attempting to take notes. Intensive patching should be avoided, especially in very young children, when there are alternatives that can achieve the benefits of aggressive occlusion without creating new problems for the patient.

There are other reasons for deviating from the standard dictum of total, prolonged occlusion. The emotional impact of forcing a child, too young to comprehend the reasons, to compete with peers with a "good" eye covered can be devastating. It is not surprising that they resist the patch. Heroic measures to force compliance with patching may actually be child abuse under the guise of good treatment.

Prolonged occlusion, even when producing the desired effect of increased acuity, can at the same time interfere with attainment of binocular fusion. This is a very important consideration when any degree of binocular function is present at the start of treatment. Patients with intermittent strabismus should be subjected to occlusion with great caution lest their binocular skills deteriorate. Patients with anisometropic amblyopia without strabismus should never be subjected to prolonged occlusion for the same reason.

Limited occlusion with high-intensity training activities can be highly effective without creating secondary problems. Brief periods of occlusion with carefully programmed tasks can accomplish as much as extended patching with little or no guided activity. These activities should emphasize directional orientation and spatial judgments as well as finer resolution and should be programmed to be at the appropriate difficulty level. If the tasks are too easy, they create no challenge and produce little change. If they are too difficult, they create frustration and likewise generate little improvement. Total prolonged occlusion depends on chance to create some periods of proper stimulation, interspersed with great periods of either frustration or wasting time.

Full refractive correction is usually the first step in the treatment of amblyopia. I approach refractive correction from a decidedly different direction, preferring to use minimum rather than maximum prescriptions and often delay initiating any lens correction. Several reasons justify this approach. It is usually difficult to refract an amblyopic eye because of unstable fixation. At best, subjective responses are imprecise. I prefer to begin fixation training before writing a lens prescription if I have any uncertainty about the refraction or if there is high anisometropia. As long as a target such as a muscle light is used, the patient can respond. The presence of blur does not preclude development of the ability to aim the eye at a light. This phase of treatment is accomplished readily at home where frequent treatments of short duration can be undertaken by the parent.

The patient is subjected to occlusion only during actual treatment, and no acuity demands are made of the patient with amblyopia. The goal of this phase of treatment is to develop more consistent ability to aim the eye accurately. Wandering fixation stabilizes and the patient develops the ability to aim steadily, which allows accommodation to become more precise. This permits easier and more accurate refraction later on. The patient is not handicapped in any way. Optical correction will be introduced before undertaking any training activities that would not be possible because of the ametropia. Refinement of the prescription proceeds along with development of more accurate ability to make directional judgments with the amblyopic eye. When treatment is done this way, there is sometimes reduction of an anisometropic difference between the eyes, and subjective refinement of the correction is facilitated. Best corrected acuity frequently improves immediately as a response to this intervention.

Full refractive correction applied too soon can inhibit development of binocular function by creating a demand that the patient cannot meet. Some patients with significant anisometropia adapt to the condition by retaining peripheral fusion with central suppression. It is more difficult to suppress a clear image successfully. Although fully correcting anisometropia can sometimes have a positive effect on binocular function, the reverse is also true. Sudden introduction of full refractive correction can disrupt fusion. I have seen instances of strabismus precipitated by optical correction, and this contingency must be kept in mind. A less risky approach is to stabilize fusion before putting the patient into a situation that may overload weak binocular function.

Temporary and/or partial corrections can be very useful. For instance, when there is high astigmatic anisometropia, a constant-wear pair of glasses can look terrible and create variable prismatic imbalances depending on direction of gaze. A contact lens correction would reduce the prism problem and look better but probably necessitate a toric lens which is difficult to fit and expensive. Youngsters who can see clearly with the better eye and note no improvement with the contact lens in place are not usually cooperative patients willing to endure the discomfort and bother of a complicated contact lens. There is also uncertainty about the precise refraction, because subjective responses are poor. A better way to proceed is prescribing an approximate correction in spectacle form to be used only during active monocular training activities. This has several advantages. The prescription can be refined and changed easily and inexpensively as needed. Because the glasses are worn only briefly under tightly controlled monocular conditions, the cosmetic and prism problems do not interfere with patient cooperation in the amblyopia treatment. The contact lens option is always available when refinement of binocular function dictates this modality.

In some instances, the patient may be better off without full correction when all factors are considered. In those instances in which there is anisometropia and the nonamblyopic eye does not require correction, maintaining patient compliance with the requirement to wear a correction is often difficult. Children (and even adults) who achieve good binocular acuity without a correction are not the best candidates to endure the discomfort or bother associated with a monocular contact lens and may reject spectacles as well. This is often the case when a good level of peripheral fusion is present and the patient does not note any advantage to wearing the corrective lens. Once an acuity level has been attained, it can easily be restored even if there is regression. In such situations a realistic approach is to monitor the patient closely, instituting brief periods of therapy as needed when acuity drops or binocular function deteriorates. This approach can relieve family problems that occur when parents are fighting continually to keep children in glasses or a contact lens and the children protest, correctly, that they note no immediate benefits when wearing the glasses. Long-term stability is a difficult concept for young children to grasp. With proper explanation that a slight acuity regression does not represent blindness and with close periodic monitoring, these patients can be managed even if they do not fully comply with use of a correction.

Still another reason to use minimal correction is related to the prognosis for a strabismus that may accompany the amblyopia. In cases with hyperopia and an accommodative component to the turn, my goal is to use the least plus that permits alignment and binocular function rather than to prescribe a full refractive correction. This approach is very useful when future scholastic demands can be expected to impact negatively on the strabismus. Having additional plus lens power available for prescribing can give an immediate boost to binocular function when needed. Under correcting the hyperopia may also lead to less hyperopia in the long term.

The ideal outcome of treatment for amblyopia is normal vision including 20/20 or better visual acuity. The amblyopic eye should function as well as the preferred eye in all respects. Consistent and permanent results are generally not possible unless binocular function is well established. In the absence of binocular integration it is usually in the patient's best interest for suppression to occur to avoid confusion. This amblyogenic factor is the basis for regression of acuity among patients with amblyopia treated solely for acuity with little attention paid to binocular function.

Long-term success in the management of amblyopia requires that binocular function be established. If binocularity is not achieved, then suppression will ultimately lead to return of reduced acuity (except for patients with alternate strabismus). Although the ideal outcome of amblyopia treatment is a patient free of suppression, how should this result be achieved?

My approach, at variance with those who advocate a strong attack on suppression early in the treatment program, is based on several lines of reasoning. First, although suppression may be the proximate cause of the amblyopia, it is not the real culprit, because it is usually the result of inadequate binocularity. This is one of those chicken and egg conundrums. Is suppression a cause or an effect? Did the suppression cause the binocular difficulty which then led to amblyopia, or is suppression an adaptive response to an intolerable binocular condition? Those who initiate a treatment program that assumes that suppression is the enemy that must be eradicated by vigorous antisuppression measures run a risk similar to those who teach children to swim by throwing them into the deep end of the pool. Some will swim; others may not, with a variety of bad outcomes. There is no need to run such a risk, because less precipitous approaches are available which minimize the possibility of an adverse outcome.

Suppression is easy to eliminate, but almost impossible to teach. It is essential, therefore, that binocularity can be established with certainty before tampering with suppression. Patients with congenital strabismus or those with significant motor incompetency may be left with persistent diplopia through the rash elimination of useful suppression. Diplopia without fusion is not preferable to some residual amblyopia.

The management that I prefer uses a cautious approach to avoid leaving the patient less comfortable or efficient after treatment than before. As indicated previously, I may not supply a refractive correction for general wear at the start of the amblyopia training. Correction is used for specific monocular training tasks, but not worn on a regular basis until there is reasonable certainty that fusion is possible. It is easier to suppress a blurred image, and sometimes suppression is useful to the patient. At the same time that monocular activities are being performed, the binocular status is explored and training activities introduced which involve peripheral fusion and stereopsis and which are not dependent on acuity. As peripheral fusion stabilizes, more central tasks that require better acuity and refinement of refractive correction are introduced gradually. Diplopia awareness is almost never created, at least not until final phases of treatment when there is no longer any doubt that the patient will be able to function with full binocular integration. Should it become apparent at any point that the patient will not be able to function adequately on a binocular basis, it is then easy to withdraw without leaving the patient with diplopia. This common sense approach considers the totality of the patient's visual function rather than focusing solely on the amblyopia. Even when full binocular integration is possible, elimination of suppression at the start of treatment can inhibit the development of fusion by placing too great a demand too soon. Patients with strabismus may even increase the turn angle because they are not yet ready to support fusion in daily life tasks.

In summary, although full acuity and binocular function are the desired outcome, amblyopia therapy should be tempered by appraisal of downside risks and of the impact of the treatment on the patient's ability to function in daily life. Questions such as what will happen if acuity responds but fusion does not, or the impact of intensive patching on the general development of an infant should be addressed before treatment. In some instances, the patient may be best served attaining a stable state with peripheral fusion, central suppression, and residual mild amblyopia. The efforts needed to maintain maximum acuity and stereopsis can sometimes outweigh the benefit to the patient. Realistic consideration of the impact of the amblyopia itself as well as the therapeutic regimen on the patient should be a part of the common-sense management of amblyopia.